The High Road to Health

A VEGETARIAN COOKBOOK

Lindsay Wagner
and Ariane Spade

A Fireside Book
Published by Simon & Schuster
NEW YORK LONDON TORONTO SYDNEY TOKYO SINGAPORE

FIRESIDE
Rockefeller Center
1230 Avenue of the Americas
New York, New York 10020

First Fireside Edition 1994

FIRESIDE and colophon are registered trademarks of Simon & Schuster Inc.

Manufactured in the United States of America

10   9   8   7   6   5

3   5   7   9   10   8   6   4   2   (PBK)

Library of Congress Cataloging-in-Publication Data
Wagner, Lindsay.
The high road to health / Lindsay Wagner and
Ariane Spade.
p.   cm.
Includes bibliographical references.
1. Vegetarianism.   2. Vegetarian cookery.
3. Health.   I. Spade, Ariane.   II. Title.
RM236.W84   1990   89-25548
613.2′62—dc20   CIP
ISBN: 0-671-76326-1
ISBN: 0-671-87277-X (PBK)

Contents

Foreword

I have a bias. I hate most nutrition books. They tend to be gimmicky, promising a "magic pill" method of dieting or longevity in a milkshake. Authors often know that the way to sell books is to say something outlandish, establishing a hook that will catch the public's attention—usually the more off-the-wall, the better. Then Phil Donahue or Oprah Winfrey call and sales skyrocket, making almost everyone happy except those who bought the book and tried the diet, only to be disappointed once again and eventually to return to their old habits. Or, nutrition books are boring. You see, since the truth is relatively simple and often not very exciting, it can also be unbearably dry and dull. Who needs that?

Ariane Spade and Lindsay Wagner have, to my delight, put the scientific truth regarding nutrition together with some excitement and fun. This is not a book for people looking for a fad diet or a quick fix. In the pages that follow are scientifically sound nutritional principals with practical advice on meal planning and preparation.

As a family physician who emphasizes wellness, preventative medicine, and self-responsibility, I constantly scan the scientific literature for new information to pass along to my patients—practical information that will help them live longer, healthier lives. Many of my patients would prefer something else. I call it the magic-pill syndrome. What they really want, regardless of the nature of their problem, is magic. A pill, a potion, a shot, something quick and easy that will fix their malady without their having to expend much time or energy on the matter.

You can probably relate to this. I know I can. The middle-aged housewife who is thirty pounds overweight and hasn't taken a quick step in twenty years buys a Jane Fonda aerobics tape and expects to look like her in two weeks. The alcoholic executive who believes he can cure his obsession with drinking by reading a motivational self-help book. The competitive runner who has patellar tendinitis (runner's knee) and refuses to decrease his training mileage of fifty to seventy-five miles per week, expecting different shoes to relieve his pain. The person who complains of chronic fatigue, high cholesterol, weight gain, and stress and buys megavitamins, knowing the root of his or her ills must be a nutritional deficiency.

The commonality here is an assumption—maybe it's actually more of a hope—that there really is a magic pill that will give us what we want. If we look hard enough, perhaps we'll find it—*then*, we will have health.

However, in clinical medicine there are certain recurring truths. Two particular ones come to mind. Truth number one: There is no such thing as a free lunch.

Healthy lifestyles, contrary to popular opinion, do not just happen for certain lucky people. They are created. People who simply expect to be healthy are often the same people who can't figure out why their marriages didn't work out after they had put little effort into maintaining them. "After all," they say, "we loved each other, didn't we?" Healthy lifestyles, like sound marriages, take constant care and feeding. Thinking, planning, time, trial and error, work, and constant effort are all involved. It takes a tremendous commitment but the results can be fantastic. But it's not free. Health, like life, is also not an end result. It's a process, a dynamic process that is ever changing, and therefore needs constant monitoring, redirecting, and renewed commitment. I teach patients to monitor certain key indicators, listen to their own bodies, improve their own self-awareness, and then regularly reassess their status and redefine their goals and directions. The ones who are successful are the ones who are willing to pay the price, in terms of effort and commitment, for their enriched well-being.

Truth number two: You can't fool Mother Nature. If there is one thing I've learned in medicine, it's that Mother Nature is awesome! Our bodies are more complex, totally integrated, and finely balanced than anything you can imagine. Supercomputers are child's play compared to the miracle of the human body. Our body's anatomy and physiology are in a constant state of dynamic equilibrium. In other words, anything that affects one part, affects every other part in some manner. Any change or shift away from the norm causes an automatic adjustment that restores the delicate balance. The body, therefore, has an inherent, built-in capacity to remain healthy. When faced with infection or injury, the human computer restores balance naturally, almost effortlessly, and the body heals itself. Therefore, when a patient is faced with a particular medical problem and asks me for advice, I often urge him to tune in to his own body's message and do whatever his body wants. Now that may sound far too simplistic, but we are learning that it may be the most scientific advice possible. An expert in the field of wellness, a professor at Loma Linda University Medical School, once said to a medical school class, "The job of the physician is to disencumber the patient from his impediments to healing!" He went on to explain, as the students scrambled for their dictionaries, that patients will heal themselves if we, as physicians, can help them understand those elements of their lifestyles that are not natural. Every time we try to fool Mother Nature by adopting lifestyles that our bodies find uncomfortable there is a price to pay. And if we want to heal ourselves, we must return to what our own basic nature would have us do.

You're probably asking, what are the specifics? What do I need to do? And why is any of this relevant to this book? I'm glad you asked.

Actually it turns out that the basics of a healthy lifestyle are fairly straightforward and simple. You know that already. Your mother probably taught them to you hundreds (in some remedial cases, probably thousands) of times.

It all revolves around our immune system. For centuries, we have known what seemed to be important for health, but medical science had not figured out exactly why. Now we are finally discovering that the human body has certain requirements that must be met for a normal balance to exist and for the body to be able to continue to heal itself and feel well. Remember Plato? That business about integration of body, mind, and spirit? He was absolutely right. The recent explosion in the science of brain neurochemistry has unlocked many of the mysteries regarding the control mechanisms involved in maintaining our homeostasis. Similarly, we have also learned how we can damage the system, and allow infectious or degenerative processes to proliferate. The neurotransmitter system in the brain controls such things as mood, energy level, fatigue, endurance, self-image, memory, learning ability, sleep, coordination, stress response, and immune response. In other words, all of the things that make us who we are and allow us to function maximally and feel well and at peace with ourselves are significantly controlled by our brain chemicals and nerve connections.

Guess what controls the efficiency of our neurotransmitter system? Lifestyle! The basics: food, exercise, sleep, love, play, and work. I told you it was simple. Yet it's amazing how many of us refuse to put proper balance in our lives when it comes to these areas. But when we do, the results are fabulous and all of our systems function at peak efficiency.

Now I can tell you why I'm so excited about this book. The building blocks of our bodies obviously come from what we decide to put into our mouths. The amino acids and proteins that comprise our neurotransmitters come from our diet. The saturated fat that leads to plaque formation in our coronary arteries doesn't get there without our permission. Colon cancer is largely dietarily related. Our level of serenity, yes, even our ability to fully realize our spirituality is, believe it or not, strongly related to dietary balance. We are, in fact, what we eat.

The truth is, the typical American diet is deplorable. We seem to be obsessed with feeding our miraculous computer as much fat, sugar, caffeine, salt, alcohol, artificial ingredients, and chemicals as possible. Not only that, but we miss lots of meals (most busy Americans skip breakfast, the most important meal of the day) and then gorge ourselves when we do eat. If any of this makes you squirm in your seat just a little, then you're in for a treat. Help is on the way.

The authors have done an exemplary job of sorting out fact from fantasy regarding the present body of legitimate knowledge concerning nutrition. This book provides a wonderfully insightful body of nutritional truth. If you adhere reasonably well to the recommended guidelines, I guarantee you'll have fewer bills from your local gastroenterologist, endocrinologist, oncologist, rheumatologist, cardiologist, and proctologist.

Eating in this manner will lower your risk of premature heart disease, diabetes, obesity, gastrointestinal cancer, arthritis, and hemorrhoids. You will feel more energetic, sleep better, think more clearly, and handle stress more effectively. Statistics indicate that you will also live longer.

Let me close with a word about a final area of concern—quality of life. The real reason to change health-related behaviors is not to lower your serum cholesterol 20 points or to lose 10 percent body fat, as noble as those aspirations may be. The real reason is much more significant and reaches to the very core of our existence. The reason to put time and energy into adopting a healthy lifestyle is because only with a healthy lifestyle can we truly become potentially who we are. Erich Fromm said that man's greatest task in life is to give birth to himself. We have, I believe, an obligation to fulfill our own destiny—to maximize the worth of our human existence.

The wellness movement has revealed a new concept of "normal man." What we previously assumed to be normal human capacities and the normal aging process, we have now discovered to be impostors of reality. Our view of normal was derived from a nation of inactive spectators with health-related behaviors typified by terribly inappropriate dietary norms. We now know that the true parameters of human achievement and the quality of life are absolutely limitless.

It takes education, planning, and commitment. There is a price. Remember, there's no free lunch. But if you want to journey into the world for maximizing your own human potential, and experience just how vibrant and fulfilling that may feel, then keep an open mind, sit back, and turn the page. . . .

Bon appétit!

—E. LEE RICE, D.O., F.A.A.F.P.
President and Medical Director of the San Diego Sports Medicine Center
Team Physician, San Diego Chargers

Preface

By Lindsay Wagner

What could an actress and a writer possibly tell you about diet or health? Why not pick up any of a number of books by "authorities" on the subject of vegetarian cooking?

This project began in my kitchen on a rainy Saturday. Ariane and I had just made popcorn and were grabbing ten minutes of uninterrupted time together. Our kids, thankfully, were intent on the popcorn. Somehow I managed to ignore the kernels collecting in the corner where they were playing "fro-the-popcorn-in-the-air-and-catch-it-with-your-mout"—a neat trick for three children under the age of five.

Ariane and I had been friends forever and now we were moms too. I had become a parent first and had two boys to her one girl, so I was the "expert" on parenting. "Lara is about to start pre-school," she moaned. "What'll I do when she discovers sugar?"

Like me, Ariane was very health-food conscious. "I wonder if I could write a health-food book," she said, "and give free copies to the nursery school."

I grabbed another handful of popcorn and grinned. "Actually," I said, "I've been making notes for a book. Not a cookbook exactly, but kind of a 'how to' for parents of young children who are concerned about raising a sugar-free child."

We looked at each other.

"I do have an education in science," she stated matter-of-factly.

"And I've been a vegetarian for twenty years," I added.

The truth was we were authorities. We were both forced to become experts because, when we started to take our diet seriously, there wasn't much accessible information about vegetarianism, or support for it. We had both done extensive research on diet and had experimented a lot in the kitchen (little did we know how much more reading and experimenting we would do in the process of making this book!). We had developed a lifestyle that totally supported our dietary beliefs. And we were both passionate about those beliefs.

I looked at Ariane. She was a good writer with a scientist's reverence for research. Moreover, she was a very creative cook. She seemed like the perfect partner.

"We could tell people about your famous pizza," I said.

"What about your ten-minute sushi?" she added, picking up my enthusiasm.

"And my meatless meatballs!"

We were on a roll. Suddenly, a little voice interrupted our musings.

"More popcorn, Mommy." The kids were back. Our stolen ten minutes were up. But this book was launched.

Introduction

For People Who Love to Eat

If you cook for anyone who is either a finicky eater or always hungry, is health conscious or overweight, is concerned about the environment or loves good food, or if you are looking for the optimally healthy or humane diet for yourself and your family, then you are just the person with whom we want to share this book.

We have both cooked for all of the above at one time or another. Also, we are two moms who take a healthy diet very seriously. Thus, we may have gone a bit overboard at times trying to cram healthy food down the throats of just about anyone who happened to be sitting at the dinner table. After years of bribing, begging, and dickering, we finally realized that healthy food has to be delicious and look appetizing; otherwise it will wind up in the dog's dish while the rest of the family beats a quick retreat to the nearest fast-food restaurant.

Indulge and Be Healthy

As the idea of writing a new kind of vegetarian cookbook began to crystalize, we started discussing it with our friends. We noticed that many of them loved to talk about all the delicious foods they wanted us to convert to vegetarian—meat loaf, meatballs, burritos, and canneloni. They enthusiastically requested lean crepes and creamless whipped cream. But, when it came to talking about nutrition and weight loss, they became downright irritable. Apparently, the topic of food gladdens the heart, but the subject of nutrition clobbers the spirits.

If you have felt this way, you have good reason. For one thing, nutrition and weight loss are cloaked in contradictions; you never quite know what to believe. Yesterday's miracle tonic is today's snake oil. The cheeseburger on a white bun with fries and a glass of whole milk, considered a healthy lunch thirty years ago, is now cursed for giving you more cholesterol and saturated fat in one meal than you should have in a whole day, and not enough fiber to keep a cricket regular.

It is apparent that the subject of nutrition carries a very high potential for guilt. It is something we all know we should pay attention to, but don't. We can't figure out exactly what to do, and when we do something, we don't enjoy it at all. It seems that, until now, the choice was sacrifice and be healthy, or indulge and risk health and beauty. Viewed from this perspective the forecast for a fit and fun life seems pretty gloomy.

But, how would you feel about good nutrition if it were delicious, filling, and satisfying, as well as an easy way to maintain good health and a beautiful body? What if meals were easy to prepare, saved you money, and even your teenagers liked them? That is what this book is all about.

Satisfaction, Not Sacrifice

It was especially important to us to create a natural-foods vegetarian cookbook that concentrated on satisfaction, not sacrifice. So we started testing our recipes on real live devotees of the modern American diet.

Our first occasion to do this test was at Lindsay's birthday. The place was her home in Malibu. The subjects were Lindsay's family, one producer, two actors, and a stockbroker and his wife. The guests arrived looking cheerful and hungry. People who know that Lindsay is a vegetarian don't always come to her house with an appetite, but this time they believed us when we told them we were cooking Italian sausages and peppers (not *actually* a lie).

In addition to Italian sausages and peppers, the menu consisted of oven-barbecued eggplant, cauliflower gratinée, and a fresh garden salad. We waited until the last minute to tell everyone the truth—the sausages were made of tofu. They watched with cold suspicion as we served each plate. Lindsay's mother rolled her eyes, muttering that the food didn't smell too bad. Then she parted the food with her fork and stared at it. We figured she was trying to see if we had hidden something *really* healthy underneath.

The producer was the first to get up for seconds. Soon, everyone was getting up for more, more vegetarian food they were conned into eating and always swore they hated. That was the first of many successful field tests.

This book contains our own original vegetarian recipes as well as recipes from our favorite restaurants and our favorite chefs. What all these recipes have in common is that they are delicious and good for you and will please kids, husbands, and junk-food addicts. Best of all, they contain no meat, chicken, fish, dairy products, or eggs; therefore, they are completely free of cholesterol. And since our recipes are low in fats and contain no refined sugars or flours, chances are you will get to say good-bye to your extra body fat. We have also presented the most up-to-date, scientifically supported information on nutrition we could find. In short, we have combined great flavors and exciting ideas with the latest nutritional savvy.

The purpose of this book is to make your transition to healthful eating and full- or part-time vegetarianism a pleasure. Start slowly and enjoy how easy it is to take the high road to health and beauty.

PART I

Getting Started

1

EAT WELL AND FORGET ABOUT DIETS

By Ariane

Like Lindsay, my husband, Leonard, and I have been vegetarians on and off for the last eighteen years. Mostly, I was on and he was off. Leonard loved meat and rich foods and his attitude about health food was very simple—if we were intended to eat health food we wouldn't have taste buds. He really had nothing against healthy food; he just felt that a few extra years tacked on to the end of his life were not reason enough to atrophy the pleasure centers of his brain. I don't mean to imply that he was totally negligent about his health. He knew he was overweight, and from time to time he would go on some heavily touted diet that promised immediate, painless, and permanent results. If you've dieted, you know what Leonard found out—diets are sometimes immediate but never painless. As for permanent, they last only for as long as it takes you to eat your way out of the depression you got from dieting. *And* you usually add a few extra pounds for consolation.

After seventeen years of marriage, our daughter, Lara, was born. One look at her and he realized that, more than anything, he wanted a long and healthy life so that he could have as much time as possible to love his beautiful child. He held her for the first time and became a total vegetarian on the spot. In the time it took to say, "It's a girl!" he went from steak, meat sauce, and ice cream to natural vegetarian foods with no animal products at all.

You'll probably want to make the transition to natural vegetarian foods more slowly than Leonard did, especially if you want to win converts at home. But I mention it so that you know that even the most committed meat eater can do it.

Overcoming Snack Attacks

In writing this book we wanted to keep the food preparation easy. If you have tried to come up with your own health-food recipes, you know how frustrating it can be. One day, right after Lara was born, I worked for hours on a baked vegetable casserole. In the end all the colors ran together and it looked like a machine load of dirty laundry. I cried and poor Leonard ate it. You can't afford this kind of experiment when you're cooking for a family that is not convinced of the merits of your new eating plan. You have to offer great-looking and great-tasting vegetarian meals from the very start.

Whether the transition is bumpy as ours was, or a pleasure as yours can be, the changes you experience will delight you. Leonard permanently lost thirty extra pounds. He exhibited a lightness and vigor that I hadn't seen in him for years. Gone were the nights of tossing and turning with indigestion from meals too heavy in animal protein and fats.

And there was another surprise. For as long as I had known him I had watched Leonard sightseeing in the refrigerator or freezer only an hour after eating a huge meal. He would stand there, with the door open, staring at the shelves and finally emerge ready to dispose of a full pint of ice cream. Then, almost as soon as he changed his way of eating to a balanced, total-vegetarian diet, the chronic hunger that had dogged him disappeared and his evening forays to the fridge stopped.

Diet War Stories

Lindsay and I know a lot of people who are always hungry. Lindsay once had a neighbor named Roberta who was always doing battle with her hunger. Somehow, in spite of it, she managed to stay thin, but she was always on the prowl for something, anything, that would keep her mouth busy. She chewed gum, smoked cigarettes, and sucked on marbles.

Another friend, Arnold, is a psychologist. Unlike Roberta, he can't stay thin, no matter what. He tries so hard to lose weight, but he is driven to eat constantly and then hates himself afterward. He likes to joke that he is totally lacking in self-control, completely devoid of character, and probably deserving of the body he has. "You can't feel very good about yourself," he says, "when you just ate two chickens and a pecan pie and you're still not satisfied." He always has a big laugh at himself, but we know how bad he feels.

Most likely you have your own diet war stories. Apart from the details they probably sound like this: At the beginning of every diet there is new hope and determination, and at the end there is the same old disappointment—and hunger. In the long run nothing has changed except that maybe you've become a little more convinced that you were created in the image and likeness of a vacuum cleaner.

Why the chronic hunger with no respite? One reason is that the most fattening foods generally contain a lot a fat, little water, and no fiber. Fat, which is abundant in most foods of animal origin, has at least twice the calories of carbohydrates, which are abundant in foods of plant origin. What's more, vegetable foods contain water and fiber that provide bulk but *no calories*. Thus, with vegetarian foods you feel fuller with fewer calories. Consider, for instance, that one full cup of cooked potatoes carries the same number of calories as only one-fifth cup of cheddar cheese, or one-fourth cup of hamburger, or one-third cup of salmon, or one-half cup of skinless chicken, or three-fourths cup of cottage cheese. You might feel full after eating a cup of potatoes, but it's unlikely that you'd feel full after only one-fourth cup of hamburger, so if that's what you're eating, you're probably overeating calories in order to feel satisfied. It's not the carbohydrate-rich spaghetti or whole wheat bread or potatoes that make you paunchy—it's the fat-filled things you put on them!

According to some nutritionists, another reason for chronic hunger might possibly be that the food that most people eat is not what their bodies want or require. Hence, the never-ending signal to get nourishment. What you interpret as chronic hunger may well be your body's demand for the nourishment it needs but does not get. While there is no conclusive evidence for this theory, there is growing support for it. Perhaps philosopher Eric Hoffer was right when he wrote that you can't get enough of what you don't really want.

The problem of chronic hunger is extremely complex and can represent a battery of other physical and emotional components. Happily, nutrition is the easiest way to deal with chronic hunger and yields, perhaps, the most immediate results. Very often, as in Leonard's case, a balanced total vegetarian diet is all you need to control your appetite and bring about permanent weight loss.

It would, of course, be possible for people to be total vegetarians and live on potato chips, candy, and soda pop. Undoubtedly, some of these unhealthy folks found their way into early studies on vegetarianism. When we talk about a total vegetarian diet, we mean an intelligently planned way of eating, based on a wide variety of whole grains, legumes (beans), and fresh fruits and vegetables with some seeds and nuts. This way of eating, with some exceptions, is inherently low in fat and high in carbohydrates and fiber and gives you optimal nutrition for the calories you consume.

Fat to Fat: Mrs. Jack Sprat

"Jack Sprat could eat no fat and his wife could eat no lean." Perhaps as a child you saw an illustration of this nursery rhyme, with skinny-as-a-broom-handle Jack pecking away at a small carrot while his rotund wife chowed down on an entire turkey.

The wisdom in this child's rhyme was prophetic. When I was in high school, it was fashionable for a girl to have a calorie counter stashed somewhere on her so she could whip it out to see if the hot fudge sundae in front of her would wind up on her derriere. "Calories in equal calories out" was the equation for staying slim. But, according to the Center for Science in the Public Interest, based in Washington, D.C., recent studies from the University of Lausanne in Switzerland and the Universities of

Massachusetts and Colorado now show that equation to be inadequate, at least in the case of dietary fat. It seems that *what* Mrs. Sprat eats affects her weight as much as *how many calories* are in it. In other words, she *was* fat because she *ate* fat, not only because she ate a lot.

The human body has no efficient means of converting fat into energy, so when you eat fat your body's first choice is to store it as body fat, usually where you least want it. Thus, except in extreme cases, the fat you eat will immediately become the fat you wear. Similarly, your body is reluctant to convert carbohydrates into body fat, and prefers keeping them on hand to give you energy rather than turning them into body fat for storage.

Total vegetarians (people who eat no foods derived from animals) are generally slimmer than their nonvegetarian counterparts and usually don't have to work to stay that way. Studies conducted at Loma Linda University, in California, show that they have greater stamina, are healthier, and have a reduced risk of heart disease, cancer, stroke, diabetes, and vascular disease. According to the July 1988 Surgeon General's Report, these five of the top ten causes of death in the United States are related to diets high in fat, refined sugar, and salt, and low in fiber and carbohydrates. It comes as no surprise that in spite of many positive changes, the typical American diet is still heavy on meat, poultry, eggs, dairy products, and processed and fast foods. (See Afterword for a discussion of fats, fiber, salt, and sugar.) According to Dr. U. D. Register of Loma Linda University, besides being less likely to acquire these degenerative diseases, total vegetarians actually have a longer life expectancy than do the general population who eat foods of animal origin.

Natural whole vegetarian foods contain none of the synthetic hormones and antibiotics found in animal products, and only about 6 percent of the pesticides and other toxic residues. In the Afterword, we discuss the problem of toxic residues in foods in greater detail.

If It's Beans This Must be Norway

The value of eating natural whole vegetarian foods became evident on a large scale in Norway and Denmark during the two world wars. Because of severe food shortages, people lived almost exclusively on a diet of unrefined grains and vegetables. The death rate and the incidence of degenerative diseases dropped significantly during the war years, and both returned to the higher prewar rates after the wars, when animal-based foods became plentiful again.

2

GREAT BEGINNINGS FOR A HEALTHY LIFE

By Lindsay

Everyone's journey on the high road to health begins at a different point. Some of you may have been lucky enough to have inherited a sense of what healthy eating is. My mother loved her family but she hated to cook. Her intentions were good and she truly believed that a balanced meal was a TV dinner. To round things out, she'd pop frozen rolls into the oven. But her sense of timing wasn't great and the rolls would invariably burn. We had burnt rolls every night. Sometimes I think the only reason I survived such a diet was because all the charcoal in my system from her famous rolls filtered out the impurities in the processed foods I was living on.

Being a child of the sixties, it wasn't long before information started trickling in about the correlation between lifestyle and healthy eating. I became aware of the terrible chemicals that were present in meat. With the determination and spontaneity of youth, I immediately became a vegetarian. I found I could live quite well without meat.

Soon after becoming a vegetarian, I was hired to do a three-day modeling job for a magazine. I was thrilled with the assignment because the photos were being shot on location at a ski resort. I had, however, exaggerated my skiing ability in order to land the job and was terrified that I would be taken to the top of the snowy peak and left there after the pictures had been taken. Fate came to the rescue: The photographer couldn't ski either and the closest we got to the slopes was a patch of snow outside the lodge.

The shoot went well. Afterward, everyone hurried into the toasty lodge for the most important moment on any location: the food! I lined up with the others and finally came to a table laden with our delicious-smelling meal. I looked at the choices: There was a platter of thinly sliced roast beef, turkey, and ham. Next to that was a huge vat of chicken cacciatore. There was also a lamb stew. My face fell. And then I spied them: cadaverous little overcooked vegetables, laid to rest on a bed of white rice that had the consistency of Spackle. I reached for them, added some limp iceberg lettuce, and looked around for a chair.

Life as a vegetarian suddenly felt like a life of deprivation. Was I to be punished for wanting a healthier diet? Was the price for a stronger, more energetic body the elimination of one of life's greatest pleasures?

For me the transition into vegetarianism was abrupt and at times difficult. Today it can be not only painless but even delicious. For starters, there are more of us today: In the United States alone there are more than 8.5 million, according to the *Vegetarian Times*. Thus, vegetarians are a consumer force worth listening to, and consequently many markets have begun to respond to our needs. In most cities there is no dearth of ranch or farmers' markets, health-food stores, and supermarkets with natural-food sections. Furthermore, if natural foods are not on the shelf, we can ask that they be ordered and kept in stock. We are the consumers, after all.

If we want to eat out, there are many restaurants that have something for the vegetarian. Fast-food restaurants have started adding salads and salad bars. Fast-health-food restaurants are even cropping up in larger cities.

Still, making the transition from being a meat eater to being a nonmeat eater may be an adjustment. Besides the cultural belief that meat is nourishing, the simple act of sinking your teeth into meat's chewy resistance has become a habit. Because of the way in which we've been conditioned, we can develop a psychological addiction to this sensation. You may find yourself craving meat simply out of the need for this textural experience.

Gradually, though, your taste for meat will disappear even though the smell of it might continue to make your mouth water. I remember one Thanksgiving I walked into my grandmother's home and the old familiar smell of turkey wafted from the kitchen. The sense memory was so strong that when we all sat down to dinner my mouth was watering. "Go ahead, have a bite," she said. My mother encouraged me, too. "One little taste can't hurt." I thought, "Oh well, just one little bite." No matter how much I chewed I couldn't swallow the turkey. The texture was no longer acceptable to my body.

But in the beginning, why not introduce vegetarian food gradually. Begin by *adding*, not by taking away. Add new, exotic vegetarian dishes as side dishes to enhance your usual entrées.

For me the discovery of ethnic foods made the difference. As an actress, my first film, *Two People*, was shot in Morocco. There I was introduced to the spicy vegetarian cuisine of North Africa. The location switched to Paris. There I met a painter who showed me the secrets of Indian cooking. He had a friend whom he insisted I meet if I ever got to Toronto. My next movie, *The Paper Chase*, was shot in Toronto! I looked up his friend. Phyllis was a very seasoned vegetarian. She grew her own vegetables and showed me miracles with tofu and edible seaweed. My work has enabled me to collect recipes and inspiration from all over the world. Along the way, I've also picked up information that not only makes vegetarian cooking easier and more healthful but can actually make the change to a healthy lifestyle more enjoyable. Here are some recommendations to help you begin that transition.

An Apple a Day

Since a vegetarian diet relies heavily on vegetables and fruits, I suggest that you use fresh vegetables, instead of canned or frozen, whenever possible. Not only do fresh foods taste better but they are often higher in vitamins, minerals, and fiber. These good things are sometimes lost or diminished in the canning and/or freezing process. If you're cooking vegetables, cook them just long enough to make them tender but still crisp. This will help retain nutrients.

You wouldn't think of putting a can of insect repellent on your dinner table. Why buy food that has been grown with chemical fertilizers, pesticides, or growth stimulants? If you want to minimize the risk of toxic residues, buy either organic produce or produce grown through "sustainable agriculture." Sustainable agriculture means that the produce has been grown with as little chemical interference as possible so that residues in the crop are minimal and the environment is adversely affected as little as possible.

Agriculture in the United States and Canada is more strictly controlled than in many other countries from whom we buy produce. Buy American-grown fruits and vegetables whenever possible and, to ensure freshness, buy what is locally grown.

I'll Die If I Don't Eat Meat

My Uncle Sidney actually believed that he would die if he didn't have meat every night. He was of the meat-and-potatoes generation. Today we know that in fact your chances of dying sooner are greater if you eat meat. Red meat, poultry, and some fish are the very foods that are the highest in fat and cholesterol. Furthermore, they contain no carbohydrates or fiber, those important components of vegetable foods that keep the intestines healthy and reduce blood cholesterol. Animal fats also harbor the greatest concentrations of toxic residues. There is a detailed explanation of this subject in the Afterword. Many people find that it's easiest to eliminate red meat first, then poultry and fish. You will find recipes for hearty, rich-tasting entrées in chapters 10 and 11.

We've been asked, "How do you justify eliminating fish? Doesn't it contain omega-3, which helps reduce cholesterol?" If you had to choose between eating meat or eating fish, you would definitely be better off eating a variety of fish. However, eating fish creates some of the same problems as in eating meat: A high percentage of the fat contained in fish is saturated, as in meat, and since fish is high on the food chain it can contain concentrated levels of toxins. Fish also contains no fiber and little or no carbohydrates. A vegetarian diet will do far more for your serum cholesterol than fish.

Raising the Dairy Question

Most milk products and eggs are also very high in fat and cholesterol and contain no fiber and small amounts of carbohydrates.
Carbohydrates, not protein, fuel the engine of your body. Stamina and energy come from carbohydrates, so don't be fooled by
commercials for milk products and eggs that promise you energy
and stamina. And, because of the high fat content, dairy products
accumulate toxic residues.

Maybe you've been thinking that whole milk or cottage cheese
aren't too bad because, as the cartons state, they are only 4 percent fat. This has to be one of the great packaging deceptions of
all time. While it's true that whole milk products are only 4 percent fat by *weight*, they are 50 percent fat by *calories*, which is
the way health experts calculate fat content. Whole milk products
are actually 67 percent higher in fat than is healthy for the average person. Nonfat milk products are quite low in both fat and
cholesterol but too high in protein, placing a burden on the digestive system and the liver. Low-fat (2 percent) milk is still 35 percent fat and contains twice the recommended protein.

A terrific substitute for milk products comes from that little
marvel, the soy bean. Soy milk has the look and consistency of
milk, and some brands even taste like it. Try some on your breakfast cereal, top your pies with our creamless Whipped Cream,
spread your sandwiches with eggless Mayo Spread and enjoy
Huevos-less Rancheros for brunch. You'll never look at another
carton of milk.

The Big No-Nos: Refined Flour, Sugars, and Oils

When flour is refined, not only is much of the fiber lost but so are
many of the vital nutrients. One change you can make immediately to get on the road to health is to replace white bread and
white flour products with whole grain bread and whole grain
flours. After you've eaten whole grain breads for a while, white
bread will taste bland and unappetizing. (See pages 33–40 for more
information on grains.)

You can exchange your white sugar for natural sweeteners such as raw honey, natural maple syrup, malted barley or rice syrup, and date sugar (ground dried dates). Remember, though, that even natural sweeteners are simple sugars, so use them sparingly (see chapter 3).

One easy transition will be from refined cooking oils to cold-pressed oils. They taste the same and are rich in vitamins and minerals and don't carry the potential refining residues of chemically extracted oils. However, even cold-pressed natural oils are almost 100 percent fat and should be used in very small amounts. You can eliminate or cut down on oils in salad dressings by using our Eden Oil Substitute (page 133). One way we have reduced the fat in our recipes is to call for sautéing foods in a covered pan, over moderate heat, in no more than a teaspoon of oil. If you want to cut down on fat further, try sautéing in a covered pan, over moderate heat, using a tablespoon of water or vegetable broth instead of oil. The results are surprisingly good. Most health professionals agree that all oils, whether cold-pressed or not, become unhealthful when heated to high temperatures, so cut out or cut way down on deep-fried foods.

P.S. on Fats

We talk about dietary fat in several places in this book because it's such an important factor in health. Too much of it promotes some of the most devastating diseases of our age as well as one of the most discouraging beauty problems in our culture: being overweight. Reducing the fats in your diet is important and comes about nearly automatically when your diet is derived primarily from plant sources.

Although the greatest proportion of fat is found in meat, poultry, fish, dairy products, eggs, and processed and fast foods, there are some natural vegetarian foods besides oils that are high in fats. For example, nut and seed butters, olives, and avocados are high in fat. You will find a few recipes for high-fat dishes in this book because they were just too delicious to pass up. Just serve them occasionally. When you do serve these foods, combine them with foods that are very low in fat.

Combining high-fat dishes with very low-fat dishes will bring down the overall percentage of fat in the meal. For example, serve Guacamole with our Baked Tortilla Chips (page 57), or raw vegetables instead of commercial chips. If you are having Govinda's Halvah for dessert, serve a main course that consists mainly of vegetables and whole grains, cooked without oils, and a salad tossed with an Oil Substitute dressing. (To assist you in creating your meal plans, we have noted which dishes are high in fats in the introduction to each of those recipes.)

Convenience Foods . . . Poison?

Most boxed, canned, and frozen foods, generally called convenience foods, are on the poor nutrition and/or high-fat side of life. All of these processes damage natural vitamins and fiber. These foods also tend to be high in salt and sugar. Commercial dairy product imitations (margarine, whipped toppings, and coffee lighteners) claim to be vegetarian products with no cholesterol, but in many cases they contain "hydrogenated" oils or fats that are very similar to the fats found in the real thing.

This isn't to say that all convenience foods are bad for you. Most health food stores and many markets carry some convenience foods that contain no preservatives and less salt, sugar, and fat. Begin by reading the labels on your packaged foods. These foods can be a lifesaver on those evenings when the imagination is gone and the cook is exhausted.

Fast "Health" Food

Many of the recipes in this book are quick and easy to prepare; others take more time. We have some suggestions that will help you create a storehouse of "fast foods." These suggestions are especially helpful for the cook who is away from the kitchen all day. Pasta dishes, such as Pasta Primavera (page 61) or Spaghetti with Tomatoes and Basil (page 173), are a quick and delicious way to solve the entrée dilemma.

With a bit of advanced preparation, you can have the basis for several dinners. On Sunday night, make a giant pot of cooked brown rice. Then on the way home from work on Monday, pick up a package of nori (edible seaweed), spread the rice on it, and slap on a bit of avocado and cucumber or carrot chips. Roll up the nori and in ten minutes you've got Sushi for dinner (page 186) and all the nutrition you need. Also main dishes such as Pecan Fried Rice (page 196) or Vegetable Fried Rice (page 197) can be ready in just a few minutes, when the rice is cooked in advance. Or turn vegetable soup, such as our Bonne Soupe (page 92), into the main course of a light supper just by adding cooked brown rice.

When I cook a bean dish, I like to make a double batch and freeze what I don't use immediately in one-meal-size containers. That way I can quickly put together Tacos (page 187) or Burritos (page 188). And you can wrap the burritos in waxed paper or foil and toss them into a picnic basket or lunch box. For other quick meals, keep tofu marinating in the refrigerator to make quick burgers and have extra pasta sauce in the freezer. Sometimes I make a big batch of Hi-Pro Pancake batter (page 60) and keep it in the refrigerator. It's such a hearty dish that sometimes I serve it for dinner with Wild Mushroom Gravy (page 139). When I do this I omit the honey from the recipe.

The Vegetarian Child

Is it really possible to raise a sugarless, vegetarian child? I was a vegetarian for fifteen years before becoming a mom. During that time I developed a way of eating that kept me energetic and healthy through twelve-hour work days and six-day work weeks. My family and friends thought my diet a bit bizarre but they didn't say much about it because it obviously worked for me.

When my first son was born all of that changed. Suddenly everyone around me became a nutritional genius. There was a lot of concern about his calcium intake. My cousin Joyce urged me to give him an eggshell four times a week to build his bones. Other family members insisted he should have three glasses of milk daily until he was twelve. The one thing that everyone agreed on was that a total vegetarian diet could not possibly allow me to nurse him and still maintain my grueling schedule. And they were certain a child couldn't thrive on a vegetarian diet. Although I was convinced about the desirability of this lifestyle for myself, I started asking a lot of new questions, possibly the same ones you will ask.

Will a vegetarian diet allow him to grow normally? Where will the calcium and other minerals and vitamins come from? Can a child get enough protein on a vegetarian diet? And the really burning question: What can I put in his lunch box that won't humiliate him when he's with his friends?

I found some of the answers in a book by nutritional expert Dr. John McDougall. In *The McDougall Plan*, no fewer than seven scientific studies are cited that "attest to the adequacy of a diet without animal products (even without milk) to provide for excellent nutrition for adults, children, and even pregnant women." The following are some excellent vegetarian sources for calcium: black strap molasses, green leafy vegetables (chard, mustard greens, broccoli, and others), yellow corn tortillas, light molasses, azuki and pinto beans, whole wheat, brown rice, and tofu curdled with calcium (tofu curdled with noncalcium compounds are not high in calcium). Other important vitamins and minerals are found in abundance in plant foods of all kinds. After all, the original source of almost every vital nutrient not produced by the body is plants.

Protein is even more abundant in plant foods than is calcium. Most vegetables, legumes, grains, nuts, and seeds provide enough calories from protein to meet daily needs. Studies conducted by the faculties of Harvard University and Loma Linda University showed that individuals who ate a balanced total vegetarian diet consumed from 111 percent to 128 percent of the National Research Council recommended daily allowance for protein.

In short, children over the age of two can easily get all the protein, vitamins, and minerals they need by eating a balanced vegetable diet. According to Dr. McDougall, children under the age of two have undeveloped digestive systems that cannot adequately assimilate protein, and therefore it is recommended that they should continue some breast-feeding until that age. Or, if breast-feeding is not possible, they should be fed a good nondairy formula supplement.

Did you know that overeating protein (eating two to three times the amount your body needs) can actually cause your body to waste calcium? And did you know that people eating the average American diet, centered around animal foods, overeat protein by this amount every day? Lowering the protein intake very often will automatically raise the amount of calcium retained by big and little bodies. This news is good for adults, especially women, who have a family history of osteoporosis. In fact, studies have shown that postmenopausal total-vegetarian women have greater bone mass than women who eat animal products.

The only point regarding the nutritional sufficiency of a total vegetarian diet that has not yet been resolved scientifically deals with adequate B_{12} consumption. Very few total vegetarians suffer from this deficiency (in fact, according to Dr. McDougall, less than thirty cases have ever been recorded), and it is not known if the few who do suffer from it do so because their bodies cannot properly assimilate B_{12} or because they don't take in enough of this vitamin. B_{12} aids the body in producing blood and maintaining a healthy nervous system. Until researchers have more conclusive information, occasional B_{12} supplements, especially for pregnant or nursing women who have eaten no animal products for three years or longer, will remove any risk of deficiency based on insufficient intake. (Note that B_{12} is found primarily in animal-based foods, so be sure your supplements are derived from plant sources.)

But back to the potential trauma of the weird contents of a lunch box. If the food looks unappetizing or strange, even if it's healthy, a child is bound to be the subject of unkind remarks. Every child wants to be normal. Enter sandwiches, the all-time normal lunch-box food. One nice thing about them is that they all look pretty similar, regardless of what's inside. Furthermore, all sorts of tasty nutritious things can be hidden inside.

But why stop at sandwiches? Your child will be the envy of everyone when he shows up at school with a container of whole wheat spaghetti or a serving of last night's lasagna, not to mention Finger Pies (page 86), Easy Pita Pizza (page 180) or, yes, even Sushi (page 186) (the latest California lunch-box rage). In chapter 7, you will find recipes for tasty sandwich spreads, lunch "meats," and other foods that will make lunch worth loving as well as eating.

The Only Sugarless Child at the Party

Two months after my son entered preschool he was invited to his first birthday party. I knew birthday parties meant ice cream and cake. I clung to the belief that I had successfully raised a totally sugar-free child. That notion was shattered ten minutes after we walked into the party. The cake was three layers of chocolate surrounded by different flavors of ice cream in neat frozen balls. On top of the cake sat a plastic boy in a toy racing car. The icing made colorful tracks all around the cake and there was a little flag with each of the guests' names marking the raceway. I looked at my healthy little boy. He was beaming. He had spotted his name.

What's a mother to do? I contemplated grabbing him and bolting for the door. Or we could stay and I could remind him of all the reasons why he couldn't have any cake and ice cream. Then we could watch the other children devour their pieces. I was stirred by vague memories of wilted lettuce staring up at me in the ski lodge. I was determined that my child would not experience healthy eating as an act of deprivation and sacrifice. I took him aside and reminded him why we didn't eat sugar in our house and that it was okay for a special treat if he had a little piece. Then I surrendered to the inevitable and watched him experience sugar for the first time.

He took a bite. He took another. Then suddenly, he stopped. It overwhelmed him. He grabbed his little flag and went off in search of some juice. This was not the only time I was surprised by his eating choices. He spent a weekend with his grandmother when he was four and when she returned him on Sunday night she told me, "I tried to be the normal grandma and offer him cookies and milk, but you know what he told me? 'I don't eat milk and sugar, Grandma. Don't you know that?' "

You can be sure that a birthday doesn't go by without a pretty cake and candles. The cakes are always naturally sweetened with far less sweetner than one usually finds in cakes. They are also always elaborately decorated. Little race cars are an acceptable part of the health plan! (You'll find delicious recipes for cakes and other festive goodies in chapter 13.)

There are many ways to involve your child in the creation of special treats. Popcorn is a standard in our house. Another favorite is frozen pops. I recommend making your own juice. If that's not possible, you can always buy fresh squeezed or unsweetened fruit juices. We always made fresh orange juice pops until I bought a juicer that allowed us to make any kind of juice we wanted. I thought the juicer would keep my kids from getting bored but it turns out they like the orange juice frozen pops best of all! My oldest son pours the juice into the molds. My youngest son inserts the sticks and places the molds in the freezer. Then comes the hard part—waiting. Sometimes we make the frozen pops a little different by whipping a little juice in a blender along with a banana or other favorite fruit, which gives the frozen pops a creamier texture (page 252).

I want to stress the importance of keeping your kids from feeling left out or deprived on special occasions. Feelings of deprivation bring about feelings of resentment, which can lead to your child sneak-eating junk food. I've always tried to be consistent with my children about diet but I'm not heavy-handed. I simply do what any conscientious mother does: the best I can with what I know. But I have always explained the reasons for my views. I let my children know how the foods they eat affect their health and looks as well as the health and looks of the earth they are to inherit. Educating your children early in positive terms will not only make them aware of their health but will allow you and them to become partners in their well-being.

My oldest son is only six but he knows what *biodegradable* means because we started using wax paper instead of plastic. He already has a sense of the connections among all living things. It makes it easier to understand his place in the universe and why he needs to respect his body as well as the body of mother earth.

The more you can distill the information in this book into age-appropriate doses, the easier it will be for you, too. And your child will know he is not simply doing what he's been told but, rather, doing what makes sense to him. Education gives him the tools that will later help him to make his own choices.

Teenage Holdouts

If you have teenagers I don't have to tell you that they are most resistant when it comes to trying something new in the food department, especially if these foods are recommended by you or are suspected of being "healthy." By age thirteen your teen's taste in food is set in concrete and the taste usually doesn't include health food. The fact that cardiovascular disease often starts in children of school age might upset you but it probably won't faze your kids.

That's where our versions of Easy Pita Pizza (page 180), Tacos (page 187), Easy, Easy Burgers (page 154), and Malibu Chile (page 222) come in. Disguised as wild-mannered fun foods, these are really balanced vegetarian dishes, low in fat, high in fiber, vitamins, and minerals. Of course, you might want to stress the fun side of these dishes and keep the nutrition part low-profile. Many of these dishes are quick and easy to prepare. Some can be prepared in advance and assembled at the last moment, which is good news for the teenager who is always hungry and also not helpless in the kitchen. (In fact, these recipes are good incentives for the rare teen who's eager to learn to cook.)

The teenage years are the years of rebellion. You might find all your best efforts going down the drain as your child attempts to fit in with his peer group and their hamburgers, fries, and cokes. At a certain point you have to say, "Look, I've told you how I feel and why. I can't stop you from making your own choices. It's part of becoming an adult." The fact is that they are going to have to start making choices on everything. They might go to sugar, they might go to hamburgers, but the chances are that with the solid foundation of a healthy body and some health education they probably won't feel very good with these decisions. They'll soon be making healthy living their personal choice simply because it will feel better.

Throw Out the Antacids

Swiss philosopher Jean-Jacques Rousseau defined happiness as "a good bank account, a good cook, and a good digestion." There's no doubt that your pocketbook will benefit when you stop buying meats, cheeses, and processed and frozen foods that are so costly. As for the "good cook" part, we hope this book will help. Now, what about digestion?

The bane of good digestion is a meal that is high in fat and protein. Then, if you eat it on the run and wash it down with coffee, wine, fruit juice, or cold water you can just about bet on indigestion. With more than 60 percent of Americans eating fast foods (and, therefore, doing all or most of the above), it comes as no surprise that the antacid and digestive-aid business is booming.

Here are a few simple guidelines, adapted from Horace W. Davenport's *A Digest of Digestion*, that will help you digest your food easily:

1. Much of the worst food-combining problems occur when you eat a lot of fat with a lot of protein. Fat hinders the digestion of protein. Almost all animal products are high in both fat and protein, so a meal rich in animal foods most likely will churn in your stomach for hours and in your intestines for days. When you cut out these foods you're cutting out a lot of your food-combining problems right off the bat, and you should notice an immediate improvement in the way your stomach feels.

2. Acid also interferes with the digestion of protein, so limit or cut out acidic drinks (coffee, wine, and most fruit drinks) while eating. This is especially important when you eat high-fat/high-protein vegetable foods such as peanut butter. Many people think of wine as a digestive aid, but in reality, its only value comes in making you a little more relaxed while you eat. Try omitting wine with your dinner and see how much more easily you digest your meal. If you just can't do without a glass of wine, drink it twenty minutes before eating.

3. Don't wash down your food with a drink, especially if the drink is acidic. Since carbohydrate digestion begins in the mouth with alkaline saliva, taking a gulp of a drink at the same time will dilute and/or neutralize digestive juices and hamper carbohydrate digestion.

4. Chew your food until it is nearly liquid. Only very small bits of food can leave the stomach, so large chunks will tumble around in your stomach until they are small enough to pass on.

5. Cold food or drink slows down the digestive process. If you have to eat or drink something cold soon after a meal, warm it up in your mouth before swallowing it.

6. Your stomach can hold only so much, so eat in moderation. If you cram it with more food than it can comfortably hold, you will feel uncomfortable and the efficiency of digestion

will drop. Chances are you will have that food in your stomach for hours. And remember that overeating is one of the great causes of obesity!

7. The points I have mentioned above apply to everyone who has a human digestive system. But everyone is unique and no one can know your body better than you. One of the most important things is to be aware of what goes on in your body. Notice if there are any foods or combinations of foods that leave you feeling ill or uncomfortable, and if there are, avoid them. Discomfort and illness are your body's way of communicating with you when something is not working. For example, although having fruit for dessert is a common practice, many people experience discomfort from eating it after dinner, and those people should avoid it. You might experiment with your own digestive system for a few months. Eliminate any combination of foods that you feel might not work for you. See if your body feels better.

Mealtimes as Rituals

In making the transition to a lifestyle of healthy eating perhaps the hardest thing to do is to take time to enjoy your meals. Turn on the music, turn off the phone, and postpone conversation about your insurance premium until later. Eating is one of life's most pleasurable rituals. Be good to yourself by eating foods that promote vitality and health. Relax and savor every delicious bite. Enjoy this journey on the high road to health.

3

GETTING STARTED IN
THE KITCHEN

Cooking is like making music or art. It's alive. It takes on the personality of the artist (cooks *are* artists) and it is constantly evolving and changing. And recipes are like sheet music. There comes a point in the development of any composition, musical or culinary, when you just have to declare that it is finished (although it never really is) and write it down.

In jazz the sheet music is only an indication of what you can do and not a prescription of what you must do. We could have continued to work with our recipes, changing them a little every time we make them (which we do, anyway), experimenting with more and more ingredients and flavors. Instead, we have declared them finished and written them down. Our recipes are just suggestions. If you take our suggestions *as is*, the results will be delicious. But we feel that the real fun will come when you allow the recipes to take on your personality, when you add your favorite herbs or spices, when you play with them and try new ideas. Our flavors are intentionally mild and lightly salted to give you the most flexibility.

Utensils

We recommend stainless steel or enamel cookware rather than aluminum, which can react with some foods, causing discoloration and a change in taste. It is also known to be toxic in large doses. In the case of Pancake Blintzes and Crepes, we recommend the use of a smooth stainless steel or enamel skillet or griddle coated with a *very* thin film of liquid lecithin (see page 35) for virtually nonstick cooking. An alternative is a precoated, nonstick skillet in order to avoid the use of any of the fat generally needed to cook these dishes. We think it's a smart trade-off.

Another little piece of equipment that is virtually indispensable is a steamer. It is a stainless steel or bamboo rack that expands to fit different-size pans. Its function is to hold foods above the boiling water so that they are steamed rather than boiled. This method of cooking vegetables is quicker than boiling and more nutrients are retained. Ideally, vegetables should be cooked only long enough to be tender on the outside but still crisp on the inside. In this way, color, flavor, shape, fiber, vitamins, and minerals are retained for healthier vegetables with much more eye appeal. Season your steamed vegetables any way you want. Try salt, pepper, and a squeeze of fresh lemon juice for a lively taste, or dried basil, garlic powder, and a dash of salt for an Italian taste.

Some Menu Suggestions

Here we have put together some dinner/supper menu suggestions. There are heavy meals and light ones, dinners with a main course and fun suppers made up of appetizers and/or salads, and menus for Italian, Mexican, Middle Eastern, Oriental, French, South American, and American meals. We offer these menus only as suggestions so that you can see how some of our dishes combine with others to create interesting meals. We would like to recommend that you begin every dinner or supper with a salad of raw greens or vegetables, alone or with your favorite dressing.

Red Cabbage and Mustard Greens Salad
Thanksgiving Pumpkin Stuffed with Rice and Chestnuts
Dr. Bob's Cornbread

Chinese Green Salad
Oriental Soup
Polynesian Tofu
Steamed Brown Rice

Mixed Greens Salad with Fresh Dill
Cream of Watercress Soup
Pasta Primavera

Middle Eastern Salad
Hummus
Pita Bread
Baba Ghanouj

Romaine, Carrot, and Walnut Salad with Cranberry Dressing
Spinach Pecan Raviolis
Green Beans with Onions and Tomatoes
Italian Roasted Peppers

Avocado, Tomato, and Cucumber Salad
Spaghetti with Tomato and Basil
Italian-Style Green Beans

Mixed Greens Salad with French Vinaigrette
Barbecue Tofu or Tempeh
Apple Baked Beans
Steamed Carrots

Mixed Greens Salad with Poppy Seed Dressing
Artichoke Vinaigrette
Dinner Crepes with Mushrooms and Walnut Filling
Carrots with Onion and Parsley

Taco Salad
Gazpacho
Tacos or Burritos
Steamed Fresh Corn on the Cob

Caesar Salad
Baked Rice with Garbanzo Beans
Zucchini with Garlic and Basil

Mixed Greens Salad with Poppy Seed Dressing
Easy Burgers
Leftover Vegetable Salad
Potato Salad with Dill Sauce

Caesar Salad
Manhattan Chowder
Twice-Baked Potato
Green Beans with Onions and Tomato
Broccoli with Garlic and Capers

Spinach and Mushroom Salad with Cucumber Dressing
Jambalaya
Steamed Fresh Corn on the Cob
French Potato Salad

Mixed Greens with Fresh Dill
Bell Peppers Stuffed with Walnut Rice
Pan-Cooked Spinach
Whole Wheat Rolls

Chinese Green Salad
Spicy Tempeh Stir Fry
Brown Rice
Steamed Snow Peas

Mixed Greens Salad with French Vinaigrette
Lindsay's Famous Hi-Pro Pancakes (honey excluded) with
   Wild Mushroom Gravy
Pink Applesauce
Beets with Watercress and Dill

Red Cabbage and Mustard Greens Salad
Carrot Almond Salad
Apple-Honey Baked Beans
Cauliflower Gratinée

Mixed Greens with Cranberry Dressing
Mulligatawny
Vegetable Curry
Brown Rice

Chinese Green Salad
Oriental Soup
Broccoli and Japanese Mushrooms with Almonds
Pecan Fried Rice or Steamed Brown Rice

Chilean Salad
Chilean Black-Eyed Peas with Winter Squash
Steamed Green Beans

Romaine, Carrot, and Walnut Salad with Cranberry Dressing
Red Cabbage with Apples and Wine
Steamed Fresh Corn on the Cob
Twice-Baked Potato

Mixed Greens Salad with Fresh Dill
Stuffed Cabbage
Brown Rice
Steamed Summer Squash

Salade Niçoise
Bonne Soup with Brown Rice
Whole Wheat Bread

Caesar Salad
Eggplant Parmigiana
Pan-Cooked Summer Squash

Mixed Greens with French Vinaigrette
Cream of Mushroom Soup
Eggplant Florentine
Brown Rice

Middle Eastern Salad
Borscht
Moussaka
Garbanzo Bean Salad

Red Cabbage and Mustard Greens Salad
Herb Pecan Loaf
Potatoes Constantin
Steamed Green Beans

Cole Slaw
Malibu Chili
Carrots and Onions with Parsley
Broiled Potato Chips

Spinach and Mushroom Salad with Cucumber Dressing
Carrot-Top Soup
Country Potatoes
Whole Wheat Bread

Middle Eastern Salad
Falafel
Tabouli

4

ABOUT THE
INGREDIENTS

ACTIVE DRY YEAST. A natural, organic leavening agent used in breads. It comes dry in sealed quarter-ounce packages and is activated by water and some kind of sugar. It can be found in most food stores.

AGAR-AGAR. A natural gelatine-like food obtained from a sea vegetable that can be used wherever animal gelatine is used. It comes in flakes or in a sponge-like bar and can be obtained in health-food stores and Oriental markets. Also called agar.

ARROWROOT POWDER. A starch derived from the arrowroot plant, used in place of corn starch. It is found in most supermarkets and health-food stores.

AVOCADO. A dark green fruit resembling a pear in size and shape. The flesh is yellow and has an oily texture. Avocados are used in salads, sandwiches, and dips and can be found in most grocery stores. Avocados are ripe when they are tender but not soft to the touch. Overripe avocados become black and should not be used because they impart an unpleasant flavor to the recipe.

BAKING POWDER. A powder consisting of a carbonic, an acid, and a starch, used as leavening in nonyeasted baked goods. We recommend the use of nonaluminum baking powder, obtainable in health-food stores and some supermarkets.

BARLEY MALT SYRUP. *See* Malt syrup.

BRAGGS AMINOS. A brewed sauce, similar to soy sauce, made from soy beans. It has a distinct flavor. It can be used in place of soy sauce, Worcestershire sauce, or any other seasoning sauce. You will find it in health-food stores.

BRAN. The fibrous husk of grains that is removed in processing. White rice and white flour are the most common processed grains. Bran, a valuable source of dietary fiber, is present in brown rice and whole wheat flours. You can also find it packaged in most supermarkets and health-food stores.

BROWN RICE. *See* Rice, brown.

BROWN RICE MALT SYRUP. *See* Malt syrup.

CHIA SEED. A small black seed, resembling a poppy seed, that can be found in health-food stores.

CILANTRO. A member of the parsley family, it is a must in Mexican cooking. It is found in the produce section of many supermarkets. Dried cilantro is generally disappointing.

COLD-PRESSED OIL. Oil that has been extracted using strictly mechanical means, without the use of either heat or solvents. If an oil is cold-pressed, its label will say so. Cold-pressed oils tend to be higher in nutrients than other oils since many nutrients are destroyed by heat and solvents. Most oils found on supermarket shelves are not cold-pressed. Look for cold-pressed oils in health-food stores and in the health-food section of many supermarkets.

COUSCOUS. A North African wheat pasta with the texture of coarse corn meal. Whole wheat couscous is available in many health-food stores.

DATE SUGAR. Not a sugar, but rather whole dates that have been dried and ground into a powder, and contain all the fiber and most of the nutrients of the original dates. Use it in the same proportions as real sugar when substituting, but remember that it does not dissolve like sugar. It can be ground to a finer powder with a mortar and pestle. You can find it in health-food stores, gourmet groceries, and a few supermarkets.

JAMS. When we were growing up, jam was made from water, sugar, pectin, and some fruit. Today there are jams available that contain nothing but fruit. Many of these natural all-fruit jams are available in supermarkets and health-food stores. Remember that honey-sweetened jams are not much better for you than sugar-sweetened jams, since honey is a simple sugar like white sugar. (For more information see page 266.)

JICAMA. A large root vegetable with a pleasant, juicy crispness. It is best eaten raw, such as in salads.

KUZU. Starch derived from the Japanese arrowroot plant. It is usually sold in powder form, but also comes in chunks that must be pulverized with a mortar and pestle. It is used interchangeably with arrowroot powder.

LECITHIN (LIQUID). Thick, oily liquid used as an emulsifier and natural antioxidant. It can be used in place of eggs in a recipe when the eggs are used to emulsify. Use a *very* thin film of lecithin on a stainless steel or enamel skillet or griddle for completely nonstick cooking of pancakes and crepes. Make sure you get *soy* lecithin rather than egg lecithin. Lecithin is 98 percent fat, so use it sparingly.

LEEK. Vegetable of the onion family that resembles a very large green onion. The flavor is somewhat lighter and sweeter than onions, which makes it perfect for soups.

MALT SYRUP. Natural sweetener made from malted grains such as barley and rice. It can be found in health-food stores and some supermarkets. It is higher in nutrients than white sugar, but like white sugar it is a simple carbohydrate containing mostly empty calories and should be used sparingly.

MAPLE SYRUP. Natural sweetener derived from the sap of the maple tree. It can be found in supermarkets and health-food stores. It is higher in nutrients than white sugar, but like white sugar it is a simple carbohydrate containing mostly empty calories and should be used sparingly.

MISO. Naturally fermented soy bean paste used in soups and sauces. Miso can also contain grains such as rice and barley. In general, dark miso has a heavy, rich flavor good for hearty soups and stocks, whereas light miso has a sweeter, more delicate flavor, perfect for salad dressings and light soups.

MOCHI (PRONOUNCED "MO-KA"). Made from cooked sweet rice that has been pounded into a paste and then compressed into very dense bars (not unlike drywall). It must be cooked to be eaten. The most common way of preparing mochi is to bake it at 400°F for ten minutes. The bar will start to melt, then puff up. Fill it with jam and be ready for a treat. It can also be melted in boiling soy milk to make thick, cheese-like sauces.

NORI. A sea vegetable, dried and rolled flat so that it almost resembles dark green, coarse paper. It can be eaten right out of the package or toasted first. Sushi eaters will recognize nori as the seaweed used to wrap up certain types of sushi.

NUT BUTTER. A creamy spread made from just about any kind of pulverized nuts and a little oil.

NUTRITIONAL YEAST. An inactive yeast used as a food supplement and also as a flavoring in soups and sauces. It has no leavening capability. It has a milder flavor than brewer's yeast and, for that reason, is better suited for use in cooking. It can be found in health-food stores and in the health-food section of some supermarkets.

OATMEAL. Comes in several different textures requiring different cooking times. Regular and Old-fashioned oatmeal are made from whole oats that have been flattened. They take up to fifteen minutes to cook and they have a pleasant chewiness. Instant raw oatmeal is uncooked and rolled or cut so fine that it cooks in just a few minutes. This oatmeal is perfect for children whose little teeth have difficulty grinding through the chewier varieties. Instant raw oatmeal is also a good thickener for vegetarian "meat" loaves.

OLIVE OIL. Buy olive oil that has been cold-pressed, which means that the oil has been extracted from the olives through pressing rather than through the use of solvents. Olive oils vary in taste from very mild, with very little olive taste, to quite strong, with a pungent, almost fruity taste. Mild olive oil, called virgin or light, is generally called for in dressings and for sautéing. Strong olive oil, called extra virgin, is used as a flavoring. A half teaspoon of extra virgin olive oil added to salad dressing that is made with our Eden Oil Substitute (page 133) will give it a nice taste.

OYSTER MUSHROOMS. Wild mushrooms available fresh in gourmet groceries and some supermarkets. They are available dried and packaged in gourmet groceries and some health-food stores.

PERO. A grain-based beverage, used as a coffee substitute. It can be found in supermarkets, gourmet grocery stores, and health-food stores.

PITA BREAD. A Middle Eastern flat bread that can be opened to form a pocket, for pocket sandwiches.

RICE, BROWN. Rice that still has its dark bran husk and germ. It is higher in bran, protein, and vitamins and minerals than white rice. It generally takes twice as long to cook as white rice and can be found in most supermarkets in the grains section.

RICE, LONG-GRAIN. The grain is long and thin. It is more fluffy and less sticky than its short cousin. It is best used in pilafs, as a bed for other dishes, or eaten alone.

RICE, SHORT-GRAIN. The grain is short and rounded. It tends to be sticky and holds together when cooked, so it is best used in stuffing, molds, and sushi.

RICE, WHITE. Rice from which the bran and germ have been polished off.

SESAME OIL (TOASTED). Oil made from toasted sesame seeds, used as a seasoning in Oriental dishes. The taste is strong, so use it sparingly.

SHITAKE MUSHROOMS. Wild Japanese mushrooms that are generally available dried in Oriental grocery stores, supermarkets, and health-food stores. They are often available fresh from gourmet groceries.

SHOYU. *See* Soy sauce.

SOY MILK. Milk-like beverage made from the water extract of soybeans. It can be homemade, but the taste tends to be harsher than some commercial brands. We use Edensoy, a nationally distributed brand, because of its pleasant, mild flavor that blends into most recipes requiring milk. Test several brands to find one you like.

SOY SAUCE. A fermented soybean product also called shoyu or tamari. The Japanese make a distinction between the two types of soy sauces, but Americans generally do not. Chemically produced soy sauces are found in supermarkets, so read the label to make sure that the soy sauce, tamari, or shoyu you buy has been naturally fermented. Natural soy sauces are available in Japanese markets, health-food stores, and some supermarkets.

TACO SHELL. A corn tortilla that has been folded over and usually deep fried. These are available in supermarkets and health-food stores. We have included our own recipe for Baked Taco Shells (page 188) that are easy to make at home from corn tortillas and are much lower in fat.

TAHINI. Also called raw sesame butter, it is a peanut butter-like spread made from ground hulled sesame seeds. Like all seed and nut butters, it is high in fat and protein. Tahini is available in supermarkets; however, natural tahini that is made without additives can be found in health-food stores. Arrowhead Mills nationally distributes their tahini, which is made from organic, mechanically hulled sesame seeds.

TAMARI. *See* Soy sauce.

TEMPEH. A product made from cultured (fermented) whole soy beans. It is higher in fiber and lower in fat and protein than tofu. Try replacing the ground meat in some of your favorite recipes with baked or sautéed tempeh. Tempeh is found in Indonesian grocery stores, health-food stores, and many supermarkets. When you buy it, look at the expiration date and buy the freshest you can find. Tempeh with black flecks is not as fresh as tempeh with white flecks, and it will have a bitter taste.

TOFU. Also known as soybean curd or soybean cheese it is a bland white food made from soybeans, water, and a curdling agent. Japanese tofu has a soft, custard-like texture and is great in sauces, sour cream, and mayonnaise substitutes and as a replacement for cream cheese in many recipes. Chinese tofu has the firm texture of moist Jack cheese and is best in dishes that should be chewy rather than creamy. Tofu is easy to digest, high in protein, and when curdled with calcium chloride it is high in calcium. It is too high in fat to be eaten alone, but when it's combined with vegetables it can make a balanced meal. Tofu can be found in health-food stores, Chinese and Japanese grocery stores, and in most supermarkets. You should follow the package directions for storage after opening.

UNSULFURED DRIED FRUIT. Fruit that has been sun-dried dehydrated without the use of any chemicals. Most of the dried fruits found in supermarkets have been dried and preserved with the use of harsh chemicals containing sulfur. You probably won't find any unsulfured-dried fruit in supermarkets or roadside stands so look for it in health-food stores.

VEGETARIAN BROTH BASE. A powder or liquid made from natural ingredients that, when added to water, makes a broth suitable to replace chicken or meat broth or stock. Where stock is called for, use a very mild solution so that the flavor of the broth does not overpower the seasonings in the recipe. Health-food stores usually carry a variety of these seasoning bases that are free from monosodium glutamate (MSG), chemicals, and meat, poultry, or fish.

WAKAMI. A sea vegetable used in adding an "ocean" taste to foods. It is very high in vitamins and minerals. It can be found dried and packaged in Oriental markets, health-food stores, and in the imported food section of most supermarkets.

WHITE FLOUR. Flour made from wheat from which the bran and germ have been removed.

WHOLE WHEAT FLOUR. Flour made from the whole grain of hard winter wheat, including the fiber-bearing bran and the protein- and vitamin-bearing germ. Because it is high in gluten, this flour is best used for yeasted products such as breads. Store whole wheat flour in the refrigerator or freezer if it is to be kept over a long period of time to prevent the natural oils in the germ from becoming rancid. This flour can be found in health- and natural-food stores and in the natural-food sections of most supermarkets.

WHOLE WHEAT PASTA. Pasta made from whole wheat flour. Look for whole wheat pasta that contains no eggs. It can be found in the natural-food and/or pasta sections of most supermarkets and in health-food stores. But if you really want a treat, make your own. You'll find the recipe on page 164.

WHOLE WHEAT PASTRY FLOUR. Flour made from the whole grain of soft summer wheat, including the fiber-bearing bran and the protein- and vitamin-bearing germ. This flour is lower in gluten than whole wheat flour and is best used in unyeasted cakes and breads and as a thickening agent. Store whole wheat pastry flour in the refrigerator or freezer if it is to be kept for a long period of time to prevent the natural oils in the germ from becoming rancid. This flour can be found in natural- and health-food stores and in the natural-food sections of most supermarkets.

WILD MUSHROOMS. Mushrooms that are generally found growing, uncultivated, the most common of which are shitaki, morel, truffle, woodear, and oyster. More and more these mushrooms are showing up on supermarket shelves, but be prepared for a price that is anywhere from five times to a hundred times (in the case of truffles) the price of cultivated mushrooms. The least expensive and most available of the wild mushrooms is the Japanese shitaki, which can be found dried and packaged in almost all supermarkets, health-food stores, and Oriental markets, and fresh in gourmet markets.

PART II

The Recipes

5

APPETIZERS, DIPS, AND SNACKS

GIARDINIERA
(PICKLED VEGETABLES)

Serves six

2 carrots, peeled and sliced
    diagonally

1 celery stalk, sliced
    diagonally

2 C cauliflower, cut into
    small chunks

½ red pepper, quartered and
    sliced

1 green onion, sliced

1 clove garlic, sliced

1 C white vinegar

½ C dry white wine

¼ C water

¼ C apple juice

2 tsp. salt (omit for low-
    sodium diets)

8 peppercorns

1 tsp. dried dill weed

Mix all the ingredients and refrigerate in a closed jar for two days.

BLACK BEAN AND GREEK OLIVE PÂTÉ WITH WALNUTS

Makes about 2 cups

½ C dry black beans (1¼ C cooked)

2 tsp. cold-pressed olive oil

¼ onion, finely chopped

1 clove garlic, finely chopped

¼ lb. fresh mushrooms, sliced

½ C walnuts

⅓ lb. large Greek olives

¼ tsp. thyme

¼ tsp. pepper

pimento slices

1. Soak the black beans in 2 cups of water overnight, or combine them with 2 cups of water in a saucepan, boil for 2 minutes, and let stand 1 hour. Cook in the soaking water over medium heat until very tender, about 1 hour, then drain and purée in a food processor or by putting them through a potato ricer or course strainer.

2. In a skillet, heat the oil, add the onion, and cook until golden. Add the garlic and cook 1 minute. Add the mushrooms, cover, and cook 5 minutes. Uncover and cook until all the liquid has been absorbed.

3. Place the walnuts in a blender or food processor and grind to the consistency of corn meal.

4. Remove the olive pits and discard, then chop the olives finely.

5. Combine all the ingredients except the pimento slices in a blender or food processor and blend until fairly smooth, but not creamy. Turn into a serving dish and chill. Garnish with pimento slices and serve with Garlic and Herb Bread Chips (page 56) or squares of toast.

CUCUMBER FILLED
WITH AVOCADO PESTO

Serves six

Serve this as an hors d'oeuvre with whole grain bread, crackers, or as part of an antipasto with whole wheat bread sticks.

1 *large cucumber
(preferably hot-house)*

3 *large garlic cloves,
chopped*

1 *T pine nuts*

15 *large basil leaves, very
finely chopped*

¼ *tsp. salt*

1 *avocado, ripe but not
dark, pitted and peeled*

1 *tsp. fresh lemon juice*

sliced black olives

pimento strips for garnish

1. If you have a hot-house cucumber, simply wash and dry it. If you don't, remove strips of peel, lengthwise, leaving thin strips of peel in place. The cucumber will look white with thin green lengthwise stripes. Cut the cucumber in half, lengthwise. With an apple corer or teaspoon, remove the seeds by cutting a channel in the cucumber lengthwise down the center of both halves, three quarters of an inch wide and equally deep. Discard the seeds.

2. Crush the garlic. Pulverize the pine nuts in a blender, mini-food processor, or mortar and pestle. In a small bowl, mix the garlic, pine nuts, basil leaves, and salt.

3. Mash the avocado with a fork and pass through a sieve to purée. Add the lemon juice and garlic-pine nut paste and mix well.

4. Fill the channels evenly with the pesto. Garnish with olive slices and a single line of pimentos running down the center of each channel.

5. Chill, cut into ⅓-inch pieces, and serve.

STUFFED MUSHROOM CAPS

Makes ten stuffed mushroom caps

10 *large mushrooms*

1 *tsp. cold-pressed olive oil*

¼ *onion, finely chopped*

3 *large garlic cloves, finely chopped*

¼ *tsp. basil*

¼ *tsp. oregano*

1 *T fresh parsley, chopped*

1 *slice whole wheat bread, made into crumbs in blender*

⅛ *tsp. pepper*

1 *T natural soy sauce*

1 *T sherry*

1. Preheat the oven to 350°F. Gently clean the mushrooms with a damp cloth. Remove the stems and chop them finely.

2. Heat the oil in a skillet. Add the onion and cook until golden. Add the garlic and cook 1 minute more. Add the chopped mushroom stems, basil, oregano, and parsley, and cook 5 minutes, stirring occasionally. Add the bread crumbs, pepper, soy sauce, and sherry, and heat, stirring for 2 minutes. Add additional salt and pepper if needed.

3. Place the mushroom caps, open side up, in a lightly oiled baking dish. Fill each cap with the bread crumb mixture, forming a mound with your fingers.

4. Bake for 15 minutes and serve hot.

ITALIAN ROASTED PEPPERS

Serves four

2 *large red bell peppers*

½ *clove garlic*

1 *tsp. cold-pressed olive oil*

dash of salt

1. Preheat the broiler. Cover a broiling pan with foil to catch the juices. Place the peppers on foil on their sides as close to the flame as possible. Check the peppers often. As soon as the peppers darken and

blister, turn them over. It is important that only the skin and not the meat scorches. Do this until the peppers are charred on all sides.

2. Remove from the broiler and allow to cool about 15 minutes or until they can be handled comfortably. Pour off any pan juices into a bowl and set aside. With a sharp paring knife, peel and scrape away all the pepper skins, being careful to catch all the juices. Combine these juices with the reserved juices and discard the skins. Cut the peppers into slices, lengthwise, and remove and discard all seeds and membranes.

3. Crush the garlic and add to the pepper juices. Add the oil and salt and whisk. Pour over the peppers and toss lightly. Refrigerate. Serve with bite-size squares of whole wheat Italian bread or as part of an antipasto.

MARINATED MUSHROOMS

Serves six

½ lb. small, unopened
   mushrooms
¼ C French Vinaigrette (see
   page 130)
1 T fresh parsley, finely
   chopped

1 tsp. finely chopped shallot
or ½ tsp. finely chopped
   fresh garlic and ½ tsp.
   finely chopped green
   onion

Remove stems from the mushrooms and reserve for another use. Prepare the vinaigrette and mix with the parsley and shallot. Pour over the mushrooms and toss to coat. Let stand at least 1 hour. Serve as an appetizer or as a salad on a bed of chopped Boston lettuce.

ARTICHOKE VINAIGRETTE

Serves one

This recipe is the European way of eating artichokes. They take time to eat and are the perfect accompaniment to good conversation.

1 *fresh artichoke*
juice of ¼ lemon

¼ *C French Vinaigrette (see page 130)*
1 *tsp. Dijon-style mustard*

1. Wash the artichoke completely with cold water. Remove the small tough leaves around the stem and snip off the spiky tips. Cut off the stem so that the artichoke can stand up. Gently spread all the leaves and sprinkle with the lemon juice.

2. Steam the artichokes or cook in 2 inches of salted water for approximately 45 minutes or until a bottom leaf can be removed easily. Drain upside-down in a colander for at least 15 minutes.

3. Prepare the vinaigrette, and whisk in the mustard.

4. Place the artichoke upright on a salad plate and serve warm or chilled with the vinaigrette on the side. Eat the artichoke by dipping the meaty side of each leaf into the vinaigrette.

FRESH OLIVES

If you're feeling frisky, homemade olives are a project worth undertaking. They have a fresh taste not available in cans. Borrow an egg from a neighbor to determine how much salt to use and return it when you're done. The olives can be harvested directly off the tree or they are available in the fall in many ethnic markets. Filtered or bottled water is used in the brine to get the purest taste.

Fresh olives (black or green) *salt*
water for washing *jars with tightly fitting lids*
filtered or bottled water *juice of 4 lemons*
1 egg

1. For green olives, crack each one with a small hammer. The object is to *crack* them, not to crush them. Fresh black olives are softer so they can simply be slit around the pit with a sharp knife.

2. Place the olives in fresh water to cover. Let stand 30 minutes, then change the water. Repeat this four times so that the olives have soaked for 2 hours.

3. Place 1 quart of filtered or bottled water in a bowl. Place an uncooked egg with the shell unbroken in the water. It will sink to the bottom. Add ½ C salt to the water and stir until the salt dissolves. Repeat, making sure the salt is dissolved, until the egg rises. When the egg floats there is sufficient salt in the water. Remove the egg.

4. Fill the jars tightly with olives. Add several tablespoons of lemon juice and fill the jars to the brim with salt water. If you like a spicy taste, add several slices of chili pepper to the jar.

5. Close jars tightly and store them in a cool, dark place. Check the jars in a couple of days and add salt water if the level is low. It will take from one to two months for the olives to cure. Taste an olive after one month. If it is bitter, let the olives cure for another month.

CAPONATA

Serves eight

Serve this authentic Italian dish as an appetizer or as part of an antipasto.

1 *garlic clove, sliced*

1 *T cold-pressed olive oil*

1 *eggplant, unpeeled, cut into ¾-inch cubes*

1 *tsp. salt*

1 *large onion, finely chopped*

4 *celery stalks, sliced*

1¾ *C fresh or canned tomatoes, chopped*

½ *C pitted green olives, sliced*

⅓ *C vinegar*

1 *tsp. honey*

1 *T capers*

1 *C water*

1. Combine the garlic and olive oil and let stand 20 minutes while preparing the vegetables.

2. Remove the garlic from the olive oil and discard. Heat the olive oil in a large skillet. Add the eggplant and half of the salt and cook, covered, until the eggplant is just tender. The addition of salt will allow the eggplant to stew in its own juice. Remove the eggplant and set aside.

3. Add the onion, celery, and the remaining salt to the skillet and cook, covered, until the onion is just tender, about 5 minutes. If the skillet becomes too dry, add a tablespoon of water.

4. Return the eggplant and the remaining ingredients to the skillet and cook, uncovered, until most of the water is absorbed, about 15 minutes. Stir often. Chill.

MIDDLE EASTERN EGGPLANT DIP

1 *large eggplant*
1 *large garlic clove, pressed*
salt to taste
1 *tsp. fresh lemon juice*

1 *T olive oil (optional)*
1 *black olive for garnish*
1 *parsley sprig for garnish*

1. Preheat the oven to 350°F. Place the eggplant on a baking dish and poke three holes in the top as vents. Bake for 1 hour and remove.

2. Cut off the stem greens and cut the eggplant in half lengthwise. Remove the skin and turn the pulp out onto the baking dish. If you are careful, you will be able to open up the pulp, revealing the seeds. If the seeds are thick and large, scoop most of them out with a teaspoon.

3. Cut the pulp into chunks and return to the oven at 350°F for another 15 minutes. Cool 10 minutes.

4. In a food processor combine the eggplant pulp, garlic, salt, lemon juice, and olive oil. Purée at medium speed until the mixture is smooth and blended but small chunks are still visible. Garnish with a black olive and a parsley sprig and serve with whole wheat pita bread wedges.

BABA GHANOUJ

Makes about 1½ cups

1 *large eggplant*

½ *C tahini (raw sesame butter)*

juice of 1 medium lemon

¼ *tsp. salt*

3 *cloves garlic, crushed*

2 *tsp. cold-pressed olive oil*

paprika

chopped parsley or fresh mint

1. Preheat the oven to 350°F. Place whole, unpeeled eggplant in a baking dish or pie pan and bake until the eggplant is very soft when a fork is inserted. The time will vary from 20 to 50 minutes depending on the size and shape of the eggplant.

2. Remove from the oven and allow the eggplant to cool until it can be handled comfortably but is still warm. Leave it in the baking dish, slit the skin lengthwise, and remove it. Save the juice. Place the eggplant and juice in a deep dish and mash with a fork until creamy. Add the tahini, lemon juice, salt, and garlic and mix until very well blended.

3. Place in a serving dish; sprinkle the top with olive oil, paprika, and chopped parsley or mint. Serve with wedges of pita or Arabic Bread (page 68).

HUMMUS

Makes 2 cups

1½ *C cooked garbanzo beans, drained, liquid reserved*

juice of 1 lemon

1 *medium garlic clove*

2 *T tahini (raw sesame butter)*

salt to taste

Combine all the ingredients in a blender or food processor. Add just enough bean liquid or water to keep the blender going. Serve with wedges of pita bread as an appetizer or as a sauce over falafel.

AVOCADO AND GREEK OLIVE DIP

Makes about 1 cup

This dish combines two high-fat vegetable foods, so the end result is high in fat. Serve with raw vegetables, or pita wedges or crackers that are made without oil in order to reduce the overall fat percentage.

5 to 8 *large Greek olives*

1 *ripe avocado*

2 *tsp. fresh lemon juice*

½ *clove garlic, crushed*

1. Remove the olive pits and with a fork mash the olives into a purée.

2. Peel and seed the avocado and mash well. Add lemon juice and mix well.

3. Combine the olive and avocado purées, add the garlic, and mix thoroughly. Serve with pita bread wedges.

SALSA

Makes about 1 cup

2 *large ripe tomatoes, cut into chunks*

¼ *large green pepper, finely chopped*

2 *green onions, sliced*

5 *sprigs fresh cilantro, chopped*

¼ *tsp. salt*

1 *T white vinegar*

¼ *tsp. paprika*

Dash of cayenne pepper if you like it spicy hot (optional)

Put all the ingredients in a food processor or blender and blend at high speed until desired consistency is obtained, about ½ minute. Refrigerate 1 hour before using.

GREEN DIP

Makes 1½ cups

For a delicious low-fat appetizer serve this dip with lots of fresh vegetables, cut small enough for dipping.

5 T whole wheat pastry
    flour
1 C mild soy milk
¼ tsp. dry mustard
pinch of cayenne
1 T vinegar or caper liquid
1 T cold-pressed mild olive
    oil

1 T fresh lemon juice
2 T chopped fresh parsley
2 T chopped chives or
    scallions
2 T chopped watercress
1 tsp. any of the above
    greens, chopped for
    garnish

1. To make the base for the dip combine the flour and soy milk in a small saucepan. Bring to a boil, whisking constantly, and cook 2 minutes, or until the mixture has thickened. Remove from the heat and refrigerate 30 minutes.

2. In a blender, add the cooled flour mixture, mustard, cayenne, and vinegar and blend 30 seconds. Continue blending very slowly and add the olive oil, lemon juice, and chopped greens, and then turn blender off immediately. Refrigerate 30 minutes. Sprinkle extra chopped greens on top as garnish and chill at least 30 minutes more before serving.

GUACAMOLE

Makes about 1 cup

Since guacamole is a high-fat food it is best served with fresh or blanched vegetables, cut for dipping, instead of commercial deep-fried chips. Or eat with pita wedges or our Baked Tortilla Chips (page 57).

1 *ripe avocado, peeled and pitted*

2 *green onions*

juice of ½ lemon

¼ *tsp. salt*

¼ *tsp. chili powder*

In a bowl, mash the avocado with a fork, or pass through a sieve for a smoother texture (do not use a blender or food processor). Add all the other ingredients and mix well.

Lay plastic wrap or wax paper directly on guacamole to prevent darkening and refrigerate until ready to use.

TAMARI CASHEWS

½ *T cold-pressed vegetable oil*

4 *oz. cashews*

1 *T natural tamari soy sauce*

Heat the oil in a small skillet. Add cashews and tamari soy sauce and cook, stirring until the cashews are completely coated with tamari.

GARLIC AND HERB BREAD CHIPS

These are a lot more fun to eat than their name would indicate and they easily take the place of potato or corn chips. They are made most easily from loaf bread, but sliced bread, even rolls or bagels, will do just fine.

Whole wheat bread or rolls
water
vinegar

salt
*garlic or onion powder (or
    both)*
basil

Preheat the oven to 250°F. Using a bread knife, cut the bread or rolls into slices about ⅛ inch thin. Brush each piece with a mixture made up of equal parts of water and vinegar.

Sprinkle with salt, garlic, and basil. Bake for about 1 hour or until the bread is crisp. Do not brown. Experiment with different herbs and spices.

CINNAMON BREAD CHIPS

Whole wheat bread or rolls
apple juice

*date sugar (powdered dried
    dates)*
cinnamon

Preheat oven to 250°F. Using a bread knife, cut the bread or rolls into slices about ⅛ inch thin. Brush each piece with apple juice. Sprinkle

with date sugar and cinnamon. Bake for about 1 hour or until the bread is crisp. Do not brown.

BAKED TORTILLA CHIPS

tortillas (corn or whole
    wheat)
1 T vinegar

1 T water
salt (optional)

Preheat oven to 350°F. Brush both sides of the tortillas with a mixture of vinegar and water. Place them directly on the wire rack in the oven and bake until very crisp, about 13 minutes. Don't let the tortillas scorch or they will be bitter. Remove from the oven, cool 10 minutes, and break into chips. Salt if desired.

6

BREAKFAST, BRUNCH, AND BREADS

BASIC PANCAKES

Makes 12 pancakes

The secret to fluffy eggless pancakes is in beating the liquid ingredients until frothy.

1½ C whole wheat pastry flour

¼ tsp. salt

3 tsp. baking powder

1 T cold-pressed vegetable oil

1¾ C soy milk

1. Combine the flour, salt, and baking powder and sift into a mixing bowl.

2. Combine the oil and soy milk and whip for about 1 minute. Pour into the flour mixture and mix until thoroughly combined. Don't worry about the lumps.

3. Preheat a lightly oiled griddle or large skillet. When a few drops of water sprinkled on the griddle bead up and roll off, the griddle is ready.

4. Pour ¼ cup of the batter at a time onto the griddle. Cook at medium-high heat until the pancakes begin to bubble, about 3 minutes, and the bottoms are lightly browned. If the pancakes bubble up before the bottoms have browned, raise the heat slightly. Turn with a spatula and cook until the second side is lightly browned. Serve at once with natural maple syrup, natural fruit syrup, or Fairy Dust (page 79).

LINDSAY'S FAMOUS HI-PRO PANCAKES

Makes about 24 4-inch pancakes

These high-protein pancakes are a real boon to pregnant women, nursing moms, and growing kids. Serve them with a natural syrup, honey, or all-fruit jam for breakfast or with vegetables and Wild Mushroom Gravy (page 139) for dinner. The recipe may be cut in half.

1 C whole wheat pastry
    flour
1 C corn meal
1 C oat bran
1¾ tsp. baking powder
1 tsp. salt
3 T sunflower seeds

3 T sesame seeds, ground in
    a blender to the
    consistency of corn
    meal
2 T nutritional yeast
    (optional)
4 T cold-pressed vegetable
    oil
2 T honey
1¼ C mild soy milk or
    water

1. Combine all the dry ingredients in a mixing bowl and mix well.

2. Combine the oil, honey, and soy milk and let stand for 5 minutes, or until the honey is dissolved. Whisk well.

3. Pour the liquid into the dry ingredients and mix well.

4. Coat the bottom of a stainless steel, enamel, or cast-iron skillet or griddle with a very thin film of liquid lecithin. Heat the skillet or griddle until a drop of water skips (it will be hot). Pour out 4-inch pancakes and cook until the top begins to bubble. Turn over and brown the other side.

PANCAKE BLINTZES

Makes 8 to 10 pancakes

Blintzes are usually made from thin pancakes filled with cheese. Our pancakes are a bit thicker, and filled with fresh fruit instead. They make a delicious and nourishing breakfast. In this case we find it helpful to use a nonstick 9-inch skillet or a 9-inch stainless steel or enamel skillet coated with a thin film of lecithin.

1 C whole wheat pastry flour
2¼ tsp. baking powder
⅛ tsp. salt
2¼ C mild soy milk
1 T cold-pressed vegetable oil

Fresh sliced fruit such as bananas, strawberries, peaches, apricots, mangoes, or fresh whole berries

1. In a mixing bowl combine the flour, baking powder, and salt and whisk well. In a separate bowl, mix the soy milk and oil. Whip with an eggbeater for about 4 minutes. Pour the liquid into the flour and stir with a wooden spoon just until combined.

2. Heat the skillet until a drop of water dances when sprinkled onto the surface. Pour 3 tablespoons of the batter into the pan and tip the pan so that the batter spreads to form a circle. Cook until the top bubbles and the bottom is golden brown. Loosen the edges of the pancake with a spatula, turn over, and cook the other side until golden. As each pancake is cooked, place on a warm dish, covered with a towel.

3. Fill each pancake with fruit and roll up. Serve with natural maple syrup, fruit syrup, or Tofu Fruit Sauce (page 261).

FRENCH TOAST

Makes 6 slices

½ C whole wheat pastry
    flour

⅛ tsp. salt

1 C mild soy milk

1 T cold-pressed vegetable
    oil

6 slices whole wheat bread

Cinnamon and nutmeg
    (optional)

Fairy Dust (page 79;
    optional)

1. Mix the flour and salt in a bowl large enough to accommodate one piece of toast. Aerate the flour with a wire whisk. In a separate small bowl, mix the soy milk and oil, then pour into the center of the flour and mix briskly. Let the batter stand 20 minutes.

2. Heat a lightly oiled griddle or large skillet until a drop of water sprinkled on it dances and then rolls off. Mix the batter well and dip each slice of bread in it to coat completely.

3. Cook until the first side is lightly browned (about 3 minutes). Turn over and cook the second side. Sprinkle with cinnamon or nutmeg or Fairy Dust. Serve with natural maple syrup, fruit jam, or Tofu Fruit Sauce (page 261).

FILLED FRENCH TOAST

Makes 6 pieces

This recipe requires a steady hand and a sharp knife with a serrated edge, such as a bread knife. The end result resembles ordinary French toast, but the first cut reveals a delicious center.

6 pieces whole wheat bread
½ C whole wheat pastry
   flour
⅛ tsp. salt
1 C mild soy milk

1 T cold-pressed vegetable
   oil
¼ C natural fruit jam or
   marmalade
Fairy Dust (page 79;
   optional)

1. Place the bread in the freezer for about 1 hour. If the bread is slightly frozen before you attempt to slice it, the job will be much easier.

2. In a bowl suitable for dipping the bread, mix the flour and salt and whisk. In a separate small bowl, mix the soy milk and oil, then pour into the center of the flour and mix briskly. Don't worry about the lumps. Let stand 20 minutes.

3. Remove the bread from the freezer. Starting at the curved crust, slice each piece of bread as if you were going to cut it into two slices, half as thick as the original. Stop one third of the way down, then, using the point of the knife, cut a pocket in the bread leaving the edges intact.

4. Fill each pocket with about 2 teaspoons of jam, then close up the bread.

5. Heat a lightly oiled griddle or large skillet until a drop of cold water sprinkled on it dances and rolls off. Mix the batter and dip each filled piece of bread in it to coat both sides. Cook until the bottom is lightly browned, about 3 minutes, turn over, and cook the second side until lightly browned. Sprinkle with Fairy Dust and serve as is or with natural maple syrup.

VARIATIONS. Fill with peanut butter and jam, or sliced fresh fruit such as pears, peaches, apricots, berries, kiwi fruit, papayas, or bananas.

SHEPHERD'S OMELET

Serves four

An eggless omelet? That's just what this is. We think it's a rather unique idea and we'll bet that no one who eats it will guess it's not made of eggs unless you tell them.

OMELET

1 lb. firm Chinese tofu

1 C soy milk

¼ tsp. salt

1 green onion, very finely chopped

1 tsp. cold-pressed vegetable oil

POTATO FILLING

2 T cold-pressed olive oil

3 medium new potatoes, thinly sliced (about 1¼ C)

¼ tsp. salt

½ bell pepper, thinly sliced

½ medium onion, thinly sliced

2 garlic cloves, pressed

1 large tomato, seeded and chopped

salt and pepper to taste

1. Preheat the oven to 400° F. To make the omelet, drain and crumble the tofu. Place the tofu, soy milk, and salt in a blender and blend until smooth. Stir in the green onion. Lightly oil two 9-inch pie pans, preferably glass. Divide the omelet mixture between the pans, smooth out the top with a spatula, and bake for about 35 minutes. The edges will become brown, the top will become golden, and the tofu will have the texture of an omelet. When the omelets are cooked, loosen them from the pie pans with a sharp spatula and cut them in half.

2. While the omelets are baking, heat one tablespoon of the olive oil in a large skillet. Add the potatoes and sprinkle salt evenly over them. Cover and cook over medium heat until the potatoes are tender, about 15 minutes. If they start to stick, add two tablespoons of water and loosen with a sharp spatula. When the potatoes are cooked, set them aside.

3. Heat the remaining olive oil in a skillet. Add the bell pepper and onion and cook 5 minutes. Add the garlic and tomato. Cover and cook

over medium heat until tender, about 15 minutes. Add salt and pepper to taste, stir in the potatoes, and cook together, covered, for 5 minutes.

4. Place half of the omelet on each dish and cover with potato filling.

HUEVOS-LESS RANCHEROS

Serves four

OMELET

1 *lb. firm Chinese tofu*

1 *C soy milk*

¼ *tsp. salt*

1 *green onion, finely chopped*

RANCHEROS SAUCE

1 *tsp. cold-pressed vegetable oil*

2 *cloves garlic, chopped*

2 *onions, chopped*

1 *green pepper, seeded and chopped*

4 *large mushrooms, halved and sliced*

2 *large or 3 small tomatoes, seeded and chopped*

¼ *tsp. ground cumin*

2 *tsp. chili powder*

salt and pepper to taste

1. Prepare omelet as indicated in step 1 of Shepherd's Omelet (page 64).

2. Heat the oil in a large skillet. Add all the ingredients and cook, covered, over medium heat for 5 minutes. Uncover and cook another 5 minutes.

3. Place half of the omelet on each plate and cover with the Rancheros Sauce.

WHOLE WHEAT BREAD

Makes 2 loaves

1½ C warm water (about
   110° F)

1 package active dry yeast

6 C whole wheat flour

2 tsp. salt

1 C soy milk, warmed

¼ C molasses

2 T cold-pressed vegetable
   oil

1. Heat water so that it feels warm, but not hot to the touch. Sprinkle the yeast over the water and stir. Let it stand while you prepare the rest of the ingredients.

2. Sift together the flour and salt into a large mixing bowl.

3. In a small bowl combine the warm soy milk, molasses, and oil and whisk until creamy. Stir in the dissolved yeast, then pour into the center of the flour and start mixing in an outward direction, taking in a little more flour with every mix, until all the flour has been moistened. When the dough becomes too thick to stir with a spoon, use your hands.

4. When the dough leaves the side of the mixing bowl knead it with your hands a few times. If it is tough and hard, sprinkle a tablespoon of water on the dough and see if it becomes pliable enough to knead. Repeat until the dough responds. If the dough is too thin, sprinkle a table-

spoon of flour on it and knead a few times to test the texture. Turn it out onto a lightly floured board. Cover with a towel and let stand 5 minutes. Since the gluten has not yet developed in the dough, it will tend to be sticky at this point. Dust your hands with flour and knead by pressing dough down with the heel of your hand until the dough is somewhat flattened, then doubling it over. Give it a quarter turn and press it down again. Repeat this procedure for about 10 minutes. The dough will become smooth and pliable and lose its stickiness as you knead it. Roll the dough into a ball and place it smooth side down in a large, clean, oiled bowl. Roll it over to oil all sides. Cover with a damp towel and set in a warm place (about 80° F) to rise until it has doubled in bulk, 1¼ to 2 hours. A closed oven that has been heated for a few minutes works well. To test if the dough has risen enough, wet your finger and push it down about ⅓ inch into the center of the dough. If a depression remains, the dough is ready. If not, let it rise a bit longer.

5. When the dough is ready, press it down again to expel the air. You will hear a soft "whoosh" as the air escapes. Push the sides down into the center and turn the dough over. Cover with a damp towel and return to a warm place to rise again for about 45 minutes.

6. Turn the dough out onto a clean board and divide into two pieces. Flatten each piece of dough down with your hands and roll out with a rolling pin into a rectangle about ⅓ inch thick. Shape the flattened dough up into loaves. Place in two lightly oiled loaf pans, cover with a damp cloth, and return to a warm place to rise, about 1 hour.

7. Preheat the oven to 350° F. Bake the loaves for 50 minutes to 1 hour, or until the top is lightly browned. Remove the loaves from the pans immediately and cool on a rack. To retard mildew, make certain that the loaves are completely cooled before storing.

GARLIC BASIL
WHOLE WHEAT BREAD

Makes 2 loaves

Serve this bread with Italian dishes. You will taste and smell just a hint of garlic and basil, so it won't overwhelm the other dishes.

Whole Wheat Bread dough (pages 66–67)

1 clove garlic, sliced and soaked in 1 T olive oil for 45 minutes

salt

Dried basil, crushed to a powder

1. Follow steps 1 through 5 for Whole Wheat Bread dough.

2. Turn the dough out onto a board and cut into two equal pieces. Remove the garlic from the oil and discard. Press the dough down and roll it into a rectangle about ¼ inch thick. Spread it with 1 teaspoon garlic oil and sprinkle with basil and a little salt. Roll it up lengthwise to form a loaf. Do the same with the second piece of dough. Place each loaf in a lightly oiled loaf pan, cover with a damp towel, and return to a warm place to rise, about 1 hour. Preheat the oven to 350° F. Bake for 1 hour or until the crust has browned lightly.

ARABIC BREAD (PITA)

Makes 15 to 20 breads

These little flat breads are baked directly on the floor of your oven, if the heat comes from below. A very large, heavy cast-iron skillet with a deep tight-fitting lid over medium heat on top of the stove is your second choice.

2 *quarts water*
1 *package active dry yeast*
2½ *T honey*
2½ *lb. whole wheat flour*

1 *tsp. salt*
1 *T cold-pressed olive oil*
¼ *lb. sesame seeds*

1. Heat the water to just below the boiling point, remove from the heat, and let it cool to about 110°F, or so that it feels hot but not burning on your submerged hand. Dissolve the yeast and honey in the water and let it stand about 10 minutes. The top of the water will begin to foam as the yeast activates.

2. Combine the flour and salt in a large bowl. Add the water slowly, kneading well between each addition. Knead for 15 minutes more. Lightly oil a large bowl with the olive oil. Place the ball of dough into the bowl and roll it over to coat all sides with oil. Cover the bowl with a clean towel and place it in a warm place to rise for about 1½ hours. Knead the dough gently for 1 minute, cover with a towel, and allow it to rise for 1½ hours more.

3. Clean the oven floor well, eliminating all crumbs and caked-on spills. Rinse it several times with clear water. Remove the racks and preheat the oven to 360°F. (You can place the racks on top of the stove and lay the cooked breads on them to cool.)

4. Turn the dough out onto a board and knead for a few minutes. Sprinkle the sesame seeds onto the board and knead a few minutes longer, until the seeds are evenly distributed throughout the dough. Roll the dough into a long log about 3 inches in diameter and cut the log into 1-inch slices. Using a rolling pin, in even strokes flatten the slices to about ¼-inch-thick circles. Place the dough circles on a towel, cover them with another towel, and let stand for 5 minutes. They will rise just a little.

5. Place the dough circles on the bottom of the oven in a single layer. Bake them for 2½ minutes, turn them over, and bake them for 2½ minutes longer. The breads will start to puff. Remove them from the oven and lay them on the racks to cool. Repeat until all the breads are baked. Let them cool completely before storing. They can be stored in tightly closed plastic bags and frozen.

DR. BOB'S CORNBREAD

Serves six

In the summer serve this cornbread warm from the oven with gazpacho. It makes a wonderful first course.

1 C coarse yellow corn meal

1 C whole wheat flour

2 tsp. baking powder

½ tsp. salt

½ C honey or maple syrup

¼ C cold-pressed vegetable oil

2¼ C soy milk

Preheat the oven to 350° F. Mix all the ingredients into a thin batter. Pour the batter into a lightly oiled 9-by-9-inch baking pan. Bake for 50 minutes or until the top is springy when touched.

RAISIN BREAD

Makes 2 loaves

2 C unsulfured raisins

1 C apple juice

¼ C warm water (110°F)

1 package active dry yeast

2 tsp. salt

6 C whole wheat flour

water

1¼ C soy milk, warmed

⅓ C molasses

2 T cold-pressed vegetable oil

1. Combine the raisins and apple juice in a small saucepan. Boil 1 minute and let stand until the raisins are plump and moist. Drain the raisins and set aside.

2. Place ¼ C warm water in a small glass bowl and stir in yeast. Into a large mixing bowl, sift the salt and flour together and set aside.

3. In a small bowl, combine the raisin liquid plus enough water to make 1¼ cups, the warm soy milk, molasses, and oil. Stir in the yeast mixture. Pour into the center of the flour and stir outward, incorporating a little more flour with each pass.

4. Follow directions 4 through 7 for Whole Wheat Bread (pages 66–67).

BANANA WALNUT BREAD

Makes 1 loaf

1 *package active dry yeast*
¼ *C warm water*
2 *C whole wheat pastry flour*
½ *tsp. salt*
¾ *C maple syrup*

⅓ *C cold-pressed vegetable oil*
¼ *C soy milk, warmed*
¼ *tsp. natural vanilla*
3 *ripe bananas, mashed*
½ *C walnut pieces*
grated peel of ½ lemon

1. Mix the yeast in warm water and set aside. Sift together the flour and salt and set aside.

2. In a large bowl, combine the maple syrup and oil and whisk until creamy. Stir in the warm soy milk, vanilla, yeast mixture, mashed bananas, walnut pieces, and lemon peel. Slowly stir in the flour.

3. Pour into a lightly oiled, floured loaf pan and let stand in a warm place for 15 minutes. Preheat the oven to 350°F and bake for 50 minutes or until a clean probe inserted into the center comes out clean.

BASIC BREAD ROLLS

Makes 18 rolls

2 *packages active dry yeast*
½ *C warm water (about 110°F)*
1 *C soy milk*
1½ *tsp. salt*

½ *C honey*
2 *T cold-pressed vegetable oil*
3½ *C whole wheat flour*

1. Dissolve the yeast in the warm water.

2. Combine the soy milk, salt, honey, and oil and heat to warm. Mix to make sure the honey is completely dissolved. Stir the yeast into the soy milk mixture. Gradually add the flour, stirring with a wooden spoon. Add more or less flour to make a stiff but pliable dough.

3. Turn the dough out onto a floured board, knead for 10 minutes, then form into a ball.

4. Oil a large bowl and place the dough in it, smooth side down. Turn it to oil all sides. Cover with a damp cloth and set in a warm place (80°F) to rise until doubled in bulk, about 45 minutes.

5. Cut the dough into two pieces. Roll each piece out into a rectangle about ½ inch thick and 8 inches wide.

6. Roll up the dough lengthwise and cut into rolls about 1 inch thick. Place, cut side down, in two oiled 9-inch cake pans. Cover with a cloth and set in a warm place (80°F) until doubled in bulk, about 1 hour.

7. Preheat the oven to 400°F and bake for about 20 minutes.

CINNAMON ROLLS

Makes 18 rolls

1 *recipe Basic Bread Rolls dough (page 72)*

FILLING

½ *C raisins*

½ *C date sugar (ground dried dates)*

¼ *C apple juice*

2 *tsp. cold-pressed vegetable oil*

1 *tsp. cinnamon*

⅓ *C chopped walnuts*

1. Combine the raisins, date sugar, and apple juice in a small saucepan and bring to a boil. Remove from the heat and let stand covered for 1 hour.

2. Follow Basic Bread Rolls instructions 1 through 4.

3. Cut the dough into two pieces of equal size. Roll out each piece into a rectangle ¼ inch thick and about 9 inches wide. Spread each rectangle with half the oil, cover with half the raisin mixture, and sprinkle with half the cinnamon and chopped walnuts.

4. Roll up tightly from the long end and seal the edges. Cut into nine slices and place, cut side down, into two oiled 9-inch cake pans. Cover with a damp cloth and let rise in a warm place until doubled in bulk, about 1 hour.

5. Preheat the oven to 350°F and bake for about 20 minutes or until golden.

JELLY ROLLS

Makes 18 rolls

1 *recipe Basic Bread Rolls dough (page 72)*

Natural jam

1. Follow Basic Bread Rolls instructions 1 through 4.

2. Cut the dough into two pieces. Roll out each piece into a rectangle about ¼ inch thick and 9 inches wide. Spread each rectangle with a thin coat of jam.

3. Roll up the dough from the long side and seal the edges. Cut into nine or ten slices. Place, cut side down, in two oiled 9-inch cake pans. Cover with a damp cloth and set in a warm place (80°F) to double in bulk, about 1 hour.

4. Preheat the oven to 350°F and bake for 25 to 30 minutes.

PECAN ROLLS

Makes 14 to 16 rolls

1 *recipe Basic Bread Rolls dough (page 72)*

FILLING AND TOPPING

2 *T Almond Butter (page 90)*

1 *T honey*

1 *T cold-pressed vegetable oil*

3 *T honey*

dash of salt

½ *tsp. vanilla*

42 *pecan halves*

¼ *C finely chopped pecans*

1. Follow Basic Bread Rolls instructions 1 through 4.

2. While the dough is rising, prepare the filling and topping. Mix the almond butter with the honey and stir until smooth. Set aside. For the topping combine the oil, honey, salt, and vanilla.

3. Oil two muffin pans. Place three pecan halves in the bottom of each cup. Spoon the topping over the pecans and set aside.

4. Cut the dough into two pieces of equal size. Roll out each piece into a rectangle ¼ inch thick and about 9 inches wide. Spread both evenly with the filling. Sprinkle with the chopped pecans and roll up tightly starting at the long end. Seal the edges.

5. Preheat the oven to 350°F. Cut both rolls into eight slices and place, cut side down, in each muffin cup.

6. Bake for 25 to 30 minutes.

PEANUT BUTTER MUFFINS

Makes 12 muffins

This recipe is from our friends at Arrowhead Mills, who make natural foods of all kinds. It's a high-protein treat kids will love for breakfast or snacks.

2 C whole wheat pastry flour

1 T low-sodium baking powder

½ tsp. salt

2 T unrefined safflower oil

¼ C peanut butter, crunchy or smooth

1½ C soy milk

4 T molasses

1. Preheat the oven to 350°F. Stir the flour, baking powder, and salt together.

2. Mix the oil and peanut butter and cut into the flour with a fork or pastry blender until the mixture becomes grainy.

3. Mix the soy milk and molasses and add to the batter. Stir just enough to mix well. Do not beat.

4. Fill the lightly oiled muffin tins or muffin cups two-thirds full. Bake for 12 to 15 minutes.

VARIATION. For Peanut Butter Bran Muffins, substitute one cup of bran for one cup of the flour.

BANANA (PRUNE) NUT MUFFINS

Makes 12 muffins

¾ C unsulfured raisins

¼ C apple juice, warmed

1 C whole wheat flour

1 C quick-cooking raw
  oatmeal

½ tsp. salt

1 package active dry yeast

¼ C apple juice, warmed

½ C cold-pressed vegetable
  oil

¾ C natural maple syrup
  or *honey*

1 tsp. natural vanilla

3 ripe bananas (but not
  black), or ⅔ C softened
  pitted unsulfured
  prunes, puréed

½ C walnut pieces

grated rind from ½ lemon

1. Combine the raisins and ¼ cup apple juice in a small saucepan, then bring to a boil. Remove from the heat, cover, and let stand for 1 hour, or until the raisins are plump and the juice has been absorbed.

2. In a large bowl combine the flour, oatmeal, and salt. Whisk to mix.

3. Dissolve the yeast in the remaining warm apple juice.

4. Combine the oil, maple syrup (or honey), and vanilla and beat until smooth.

5. Stir the plumped raisins, bananas (or prunes), walnuts, and lemon rind into the maple syrup mixture. Add the dissolved yeast and stir well.

6. Add the liquid ingredients to the flour and stir well. Oil 12 muffin cups and fill each one three-quarters full. Let stand in a warm place for 10 minutes.

7. Preheat the oven to 400°F and bake for 25 minutes or until a clean probe inserted into the center of a muffin comes out clean.

VARIATIONS. For Banana (Prune) Nut Bran Muffins substitute one cup of bran for one cup of the flour.

For Filled Banana (Prune) Nut Muffins prepare muffin dough as indicated. Fill muffin cups halfway. Place one teaspoon of jam or prune spread in the center of each cup and cover with the remainder of the dough. Bake as directed.

BAKER'S DOZEN MUFFINS

Makes 13 muffins

Try as we might to get this recipe to make twelve muffins, we always wind up with an extra muffin, a baker's dozen. So, unless you have an old-fashioned muffin pan that turns out great big muffins, use one double or two regular muffin pans and a custard cup for the extra muffin.

¾ C unsulfured raisins

¼ C apple juice

1 C whole wheat pastry flour

1 C quick-cooking raw oatmeal

3½ tsp. baking powder

½ tsp. salt

3 T date sugar (ground dried dates)

2 T cold-pressed vegetable oil

3 T honey

¼ tsp. cream of tartar

2 tsp. natural vanilla

1¾ C soy milk

1 tsp. fresh lemon juice

¾ C chopped walnuts

1. Combine the raisins and apple juice in a small saucepan and bring to a boil. Remove from the heat, cover, and let stand until the raisins are plump, about 1 hour.

2. In a mixing bowl, combine the flour, oatmeal, baking powder, salt, and date sugar. Whisk well to mix.

3. In a separate bowl, combine the oil, honey, cream of tartar, vanilla, soy milk, and lemon juice. Beat with an eggbeater until the mixture is frothy, about 5 minutes, then slowly pour into the flour, stirring gently until completely combined. Gently stir in the walnuts. The mixture will be rather lumpy. Do not overstir to make a smooth batter or the muffins will be tough.

4. Pour into oiled muffin pans. Preheat the oven to 400°F and bake for 20 minutes or until a clean probe inserted into the corner of one muffin comes out clean.

VARIATIONS. To make Bran Muffins substitute one cup of bran for the oatmeal.

For Filled Muffins prepare muffin batter as indicated. Fill muffin cups halfway. Place one teaspoon of jam or prune spread in the center of each cup and cover with the remainder of the batter. Bake as directed.

APPLE-APRICOT STRUDEL

Strudel dough should be rolled out very thin and the ingredients should be juicy. Thus, transferring the strudel, unbroken, onto the baking sheet is very difficult. For this reason we recommend that you make two smaller, easy-to-handle strudels, instead of one big one.

DOUGH

1½ C whole wheat pastry flour

¼ tsp. salt

1 T oil

⅓ to ½ C water

1 tsp. vinegar

FILLING

½ C unsulfured raisins

3 T apple juice

½ C chopped unsulfured dried apricots

2 medium-tart apples

2 T date sugar (ground dried dates)

½ C chopped walnuts

cold-pressed vegetable oil

1. To make the dough, mix the flour and the salt in a mixing bowl. Whisk together the oil, water, and vinegar. Start by using ⅓ cup of water and add more water as necessary. Make a well in the flour and pour the liquid ingredients into it. Blend the flour into the liquid. This job is a little easier (although messier) if you use your hands. The dough should be soft and a little sticky, but not wet. If it is too dry, add more water, a little at a time. Knead the dough for about 10 minutes, cover with a warm bowl, and set aside for 45 minutes.

2. To make the filling, place the raisins and apricots in a small sauce-pan with the apple juice, bring to a boil, and cook, covered, for 3 minutes.

3. Peel the apples and cut each one into eight wedges, then cut crosswise into medium-thin slices.

4. Cut the dough into two equal pieces. Place the first on a large piece of lightly floured waxed paper. Roll out very thin, but not so thin that it starts falling apart. After each rolling, very gently separate the dough from the waxed paper to prevent sticking. Dip your fingers in a little oil and very lightly oil the dough, leaving ¾ inch around the edges unoiled. Sprinkle half of the

date sugar, raisins, apples, walnuts, and apricots over the dough, leaving the same ¾-inch border. Roll up the dough, starting with the longer side. Moisten the seams with a little water and seal. Lift up the waxed paper and roll the strudel onto a lightly oiled baking sheet. Repeat for the second strudel.

5. Brush the tops very lightly with a mixture of oil and water, especially where there is loose flour. Preheat the oven to 400°F and bake for 30 minutes. Reduce heat to 350°F and bake for 10 minutes more.

FAIRY DUST

Sprinkle on French toast, pancakes, toast with peanut butter, or fresh fruit.

¼ C grated dried coconut

¼ C date sugar (powdered dried dates)

Mix the coconut and date sugar in a mortar and pestle and grind into a fine powder.

MUESLI

Makes 2½ cups

This breakfast cereal first came from Switzerland. The light toasting of the oatmeal makes it easier to chew and digest. Try adding your own combinations of nuts, seeds, and fresh fruit.

2 C quick-cooking raw oatmeal

½ C chopped unsulfured dried fruits (such as raisins, dates, prunes, pineapple, mango, papaya)

2 T dry-roasted sunflower seeds, hulled

1 T oat bran (optional)

1. Heat the oatmeal in a skillet until it becomes slightly golden, then remove from the skillet immediately. Browning it will impart a bitter taste.

2. Mix all the ingredients in a bowl and serve with soy milk and a generous helping of fresh fruit.

7

SANDWICHES, SPREADS, AND LUNCH BOX GOODIES

PEANUT BUTTER AND BANANA SANDWICH

Serves one

Legend has it that Elvis Presley's favorite sandwich was peanut butter and bananas, deep fried. For obvious reasons we have omitted the deep frying, and invite you to make the sandwich on toast, instead. It will probably become a lunch box favorite.

1 *T natural peanut butter*
2 *slices whole wheat bread*
   (toasted, if desired)

½ *banana, ripe but not dark*
cinnamon or *nutmeg*
   (optional)

Spread the peanut butter on one piece of bread. Peel a banana, slice it, and cover the peanut butter with the slices. Sprinkle with cinnamon or nutmeg if desired. Top with a second piece of bread and cut in half.

Vegetarian "Salami"

Makes 1 pound (24 slices)

We really didn't know what to call this. It is a delicious alternative to spiced meats such as salami, bologna, or corned beef.

1 lb. firm Chinese-style tofu
1 quart water
Tempeh Marinade (page 143)

1 garlic clove, thinly sliced
⅛ tsp. ground black pepper.

1. Drain the tofu and slice it into four equal pieces. Place the tofu and water in a saucepan, bring to a boil, and cook for 7 minutes. Drain and cut into slices about ⅛ inch thick. Lay slices in one layer on a clean, thick kitchen towel. Cover with another thick kitchen towel and lay some heavy books on top to press out the water. Let stand for 30 minutes.

2. Prepare the Tofu Marinade and add the garlic and black pepper to it at the end. Pour a little marinade into a flat-bottomed container that has a lid that seals and lay one layer of tofu in it. Cover with marinade and add another layer of tofu. Repeat until all the tofu and marinade are used up. Refrigerate for two days. If the marinade does not cover the tofu, turn container upside-down for half the time. The tofu can remain in the marinade for up to four days. The longer it soaks, the stronger it will be. If you prefer the slices to be drier, remove them from the marinade and lay them in one layer on a dish in the refrigerator for several hours. After the tofu has been removed from the marinade, store it wrapped or covered in the refrigerator for up to two days, or wrap tightly and freeze.

3. Use in sandwiches as you would use cold cuts, or cut up in salads.

REUBEN SANDWICH

Makes one sandwich

1 T Russian Dressing (page 131)

2 slices rye bread

2 slices Vegetarian "Salami" (page 82)

3 T sauerkraut, or 3 T coleslaw and dill pickle slices

Prepare the Russian Dressing and preheat the oven to 400°F. Spread half of the Russian Dressing on one side of one piece of bread. Add the slices of Vegetarian "Salami," and cover with sauerkraut or coleslaw and pickles. Spread the remainder of the Russian Dressing on top. Cover with the second piece of bread and bake for 5 minutes until heated through.

HAWAIIAN SANDWICH

Makes one sandwich

2 slices whole wheat bread

Chinese mustard (Dijon mustard can be used)

2 slices Vegetarian "Salami" (page 82)

2 slices fresh or water-packed canned pineapple

½ tsp. chopped chives

Spread both slices of bread with Chinese mustard. Cover one slice with the Vegetarian "Salami" and pineapple slices. Sprinkle the chives on top. Cover with the second piece of bread and cut in half diagonally.

FALAFEL

Makes 16 patties

Real Middle Eastern falafel is usually spicy-hot enough to blow off your ears. Feel free to add as much or as little cayenne pepper as your constitution can stand. Also we have omitted the deep frying in favor of broiling.

FALAFEL

3 C boiling water

½ C raw dried yellow split peas

½ C raw garbanzo beans

¼ to ½ tsp. salt

½ tsp. black pepper

1 T chopped fresh parsley

¼ tsp. garlic powder

¾ tsp. ground cumin

¼ tsp. onion powder

dash of cayenne (optional)

SANDWICH

pita bread

falafel patties

tomato wedges

shredded lettuce

chopped green onions

chopped parsley

Hummus (page 52), thinned with enough water to make a sauce (replace some of the water with vinegar for a piquant taste)

1. To make the falafel, pour the boiling water over the split peas and garbanzo beans, cover, and let stand for 1½ hours. Drain and reserve the soaking water. Place the peas and beans in a food processor or blender and at high speed blend until they are the same consistency as damp, coarse corn meal. Add all the other falafel ingredients and blend enough to mix well. Add enough soaking liquid so that the mixture feels wet, about ½ cup. Add the liquid ¼ cup at a time. The patties should be wet but still hold together. A drier raw patty will result in a harder cooked patty.

2. Form the mixture into tightly packed patties 1½ inches across and about ⅔ inch thick. Stack them on a steaming tray and stream for 30 minutes. Check the level of the steaming water and add some if it starts to run dry. The patties can be wrapped and frozen at this point.

3. Place the steamed patties on a baking sheet and broil 6 inches from the heat until lightly browned. Turn over and brown the second side.

Broiler heats vary, but 5 minutes on each side should do the trick.

4. To make sandwiches, cut the pita breads in two. Open up the pocket and fill with two or three falafel patties, depending on the size of the pita, two or three tomato wedges, and shredded lettuce. Sprinkle with chopped onions and parsley and cover the stuffing with a generous portion of thinned Hummus sauce.

WATERCRESS AND CUCUMBER SANDWICH

Makes one sandwich

Try this sandwich on a hot summer day along with a frosty glass of iced mint tea.

2 *slices whole wheat bread (can be toasted)*

Mayo Spread I (page 87) or mayonnaise

Dijon mustard

10 *thin slices of cucumber*

3 *large sprigs watercress, washed and stems removed*

2 *slices of tomato*

Spread one side of the bread with mayonnaise and mustard. On one piece, lay out a double layer of cucumber. Follow with a generous covering of the watercress and tomato and cover with the second piece of bread. Cut diagonally.

FINGER PIES

Makes 18 pies

Lunch boxes never had it so good. These easy-to-make little treats can be filled with Pecan Fried Rice (page 196), Apple-Honey Baked Beans, (page 223), Malibu Chile (page 222), or steamed veggies. Part of the fun of eating these neat little packages is discovering what's inside.

2 *C whole wheat pastry
    flour (cold)*

¼ *tsp. salt*

5 *T cold-pressed vegetable
    oil (cold)*

5 to 8 *T ice water*

1 *C filling of your choice*

1. Whisk the flour and salt together. Cut the oil into the flour until the flour is the consistency of corn grits. Slowly sprinkle the water onto the dough, stirring quickly. The dough should form easily into a ball and should not be sticky.

2. Cover the dough and let stand 10 minutes. Cut the dough into two equal pieces. Place each piece between two pieces of waxed paper and roll out into a rectangle about ⅛ inch thick. Cut into thirds and then turn and cut into thirds again, forming nine, approximately equal, rectangles. Place 1 tablespoon of filling on one side of each rectangle, fold over, and press down on each seam with a fork to seal.

3. Preheat the oven to 350°F and bake for 20 minutes. For fruit-filled Finger Pies, see chapter 13.

MAYO SPREAD I

Makes about 1⅔ cups

Regular mayonnaise is about 99 percent fat and provides a whopping 11.2 grams of fat per tablespoon. Even the low-fat variety contains 5 grams of fat. This dressing, which tastes and spreads like real mayonnaise, contains just 1.08 grams of fat per tablespoon. Use chilled Mayo Spread as mayonnaise in salad dressings and as a sandwich spread.

5 *T whole wheat pastry flour*	*pinch of cayenne*
1 *C water*	1 *T vinegar* or *caper liquid*
½ *tsp. salt*	2 *T cold-pressed vegetable oil*
¼ *tsp. dry mustard*	1 *T fresh lemon juice*

1. Pass the flour through a tea strainer to remove the course bran. Combine the flour and water in a small saucepan and bring to a boil, whisking constantly. Cook for two minutes, until the mixture thickens. Cool to room temperature.

2. Place the cooled flour mixture in a blender along with the salt, mustard, cayenne, and half of the vinegar. Turn on the blender to medium speed and very slowly add the oil. Add the lemon juice and the rest of the vinegar and blend just enough to mix. Turn the blender off immediately. Refrigerate.

MAYO SPREAD II

Makes 2½ cups

Mayo Spread II is lighter than Mayo Spread I and has even less fat: .88 grams per tablespoon. The fat can be further reduced to .53 grams per tablespoon by reducing the oil as indicated.

½ C water

1 T plus 1 tsp. agar flakes

1 tsp. arrowroot powder

1¼ C mild soy milk

¼ tsp. dry mustard

½ to 1 tsp. salt

dash of cayenne pepper

1½ T white vinegar

2 T cold-pressed olive oil
(can be reduced to 1 T
for fat-restricted diets)

1 T fresh lemon juice

1. Place the water and agar flakes in a small saucepan, bring to a boil, and simmer for 6 minutes, stirring often.

2. Dissolve the arrowroot powder in 1 tablespoon of the soy milk. Add it to the simmering agar mixture, whisking briskly. Cook 2 minutes more or until the mixture thickens.

3. Pour the soy milk into a blender and turn it on. Slowly add the agar mixture. Add the dry mustard, salt, cayenne, and vinegar. Very slowly add the olive oil. Add the lemon juice and turn the blender off immediately. Refrigerate for 1 hour. Can be stored in a closed container in the refrigerator for several weeks.

BREAD SPREAD

Makes 1½ cups

This spread is our low-fat answer to butter. If you substitute clarified butter for the oil, the spread will have a buttery taste.

5 T whole wheat pastry
    flour
1 C water

⅛ tsp. salt
1½ T cold-pressed vegetable
    oil

1. Pass the flour through a tea strainer to remove the coarse bran. In a small saucepan, mix the flour and water and bring to a boil, whisking constantly. If clumps appear, beat smooth with an eggbeater. Cook approximately 2 minutes or until thickened. Cool 10 minutes.

2. Combine all the ingredients in a blender and blend at medium speed until smooth. Chill and use just as you would butter on bread and crackers and steamed vegetables. This spread cannot, however, be used in place of butter for cooking or baking.

CASHEW BUTTER

Makes 1¾ cups

Cashew and almond butters are a nice change when peanut butter has worn out its welcome. Cashew and almond butter sandwiches with jam can appear where peanut butter sandwiches wouldn't dare, such as at luncheons and high teas. They have a delicate flavor and an elegantly light color.

2 C raw cashew pieces

2⅓ T cold-pressed vegetable oil

Place the cashews in a blender and grind them into a meal at medium speed. Add the oil and blend until creamy, about 5 minutes. If the

cashew butter is going to be used as a spread, salt can be added to taste. Do not add salt is you intend to use the butter in cooking.

Almond Butter

Makes 1¾ cups

2 C raw almonds, blanched
or with skins

2⅓ C cold-pressed vegetable
oil

Follow the directions for Cashew Butter (page 89). However, almonds are much harder so it is helpful to heat the oil slightly before adding it.

It might be necessary to turn the blender off and wait a minute or so if the motor starts to heat up.

Prune Spread

Makes 1 cup

20 unsulfured pitted or
unpitted prunes

apple juice
grated peel of ½ lemon

Place the prunes in a small saucepan with just enough apple juice to cover. Boil 5 minutes, then let stand, covered, for 2 hours. If the prunes are not pitted, remove the pits. Pu-

rée the prunes in a blender with the lemon peel. Add enough of the soaking liquid to make a creamy paste. Serve in place of jam.

8

SOUPS

BORSCHT

Makes 8 cups

This soup is traditional in Russia where it is served either hot or cold.

4 *large beets with greens and stems*

6 *C broth or stock (or 2 T natural soy sauce in 6 C water)*

1 *onion, chopped finely*

1 *large carrot, chopped finely*

1½ *C chopped red cabbage*

4 *T white vinegar (or more if you like it piquant)*

½ *tsp. caraway seeds*

1 *T honey*

1. Wash the beets with their stems and leaves and remove the roots. Remove any leaves or stems that are wilted. Chop the beets, stems, and leaves. A food processor is a real timesaver for this job. Bring 2 cups of the broth or water with soy sauce to a boil in a 9-quart saucepan. Add beets, onion, and carrot and cook, covered, over medium heat for 20 minutes.

2. Add cabbage, vinegar, caraway seeds, and remainder of broth or water with soy sauce. Bring to a boil and cook 30 minutes more. Water may be added to make a lighter soup. Remove from heat and stir in the honey. To serve cold, add thin slices of cucumber, Avocado Sour Cream (page 135), or Tofu Sour Cream (page 134). To serve hot, add a boiled baby potato or rye bread Croutons (page 119).

BONNE SOUPE

Serves six

This means, literally, "good soup" in French. It's practically a staple in the French countryside, and it's usually made out of whatever winter vegetables are available.

2 *large potatoes, cubed*

3 *large carrots, sliced*

½ *lb. winter squash, peeled, seeds removed, cubed (Any kind will do including pumpkin, acorn, banana, and turban.)*

1 *leek, finely chopped*

½ *lb. fresh green beans, strings removed and cut into 1-inch sections*

½ *C fresh peas (Use frozen peas if fresh are not available.)*

1 *T chopped fresh parsley*

1 *tsp. salt*

½ *tsp. pepper*

Place all the ingredients in a large kettle, add water to cover, and bring to a boil. Turn down heat and simmer for 30 minutes. Remove half of the soup, mash thoroughly using potato ricer, food processor, or blender, and return to the rest of the soup. Serve hot with warm bread.

CARROT-TOP SOUP

Serves six

Take a large bowl of Carrot-Top Soup, a fresh loaf of whole wheat bread, and a pair of warm old slippers and you have all you need to make a cold winter evening cozy and satisfying.

1 C black-eyed peas, soaked
    overnight

½ C dried split peas

½ C pearl barley

3 quarts water

1 T cold-pressed olive oil

½ large onion, chopped

2 medium carrots, sliced

4 carrot tops (greens only,
    stems removed),
    chopped

2 large mustard greens,
    chopped

1 leek, sliced

1 C green beans, broken
    into 1-inch sections

1 large potato, unpeeled,
    diced

½ bay leaf

¼ tsp. thyme

¼ tsp. tarragon

¼ tsp. savory

1 tsp. salt

dash pepper

1. In a large pot, place the black-eyed peas, split peas, pearl barley, and water and simmer until the beans are tender, about 45 minutes.

2. In a skillet heat the olive oil. Add the onions and sauté, covered, 10 minutes or until the onions begin to brown. Turn off the heat under the onions and pour about ½ C of the bean cooking water into the skillet and mix well.

3. When the beans are cooked, add the onions and all the other ingredients to the bean pot and cook another 30 minutes, or until the vegetables are tender. Serve in large soup bowls with generous servings of fresh whole wheat or black bread.

CREAM OF WATERCRESS SOUP

Serves six

2 tsp. cold-pressed olive oil

2 onions, finely chopped

1 clove garlic, finely chopped

3 large baking potatoes, very thinly sliced

½ C water

¼ tsp. ground black pepper

1 tsp. salt

1 bunch watercress

1 C soy or almond milk

½ C water

1. Heat the oil in a large saucepan. Sauté the onions, covered, until transparent. Add the garlic and sauté for 1 minute more. Add the potatoes, water, pepper, and salt, cover, and bring to a boil. Reduce and cook, covered, until the potatoes break apart when stirred, about 15 minutes. It is important to have a minimum amount of water in the pot, so check it often to make sure the potatoes don't burn. If the potatoes start to stick, remove them from the heat for 1 minute, stir, and return to heat.

2. Wash the watercress and set aside six small sprigs for garnish. Cut up the rest, stems included, and add to the potatoes along with the soy milk and additional water.

3. Place the soup in a blender or food processor and blend at medium speed until very smooth and creamy, about 5 minutes. Return soup to the saucepan and cook for 5 minutes. Garnish with watercress sprigs and serve.

CREAM OF MUSHROOM SOUP

Serves six

2 tsp. cold-pressed olive oil

2 onions, chopped

1 stalk of celery, sliced

1 clove garlic

3 large baking potatoes, very thinly sliced

½ C water

¼ tsp. ground black pepper

1 tsp. salt

¼ lb. small mushrooms, sliced

1 C soy milk

½ C water

1. Heat the oil in a large saucepan and sauté the onions until golden. Add the celery and garlic and cook for 5 minutes. Add the potatoes, water, pepper, and salt and bring to a boil. Reduce heat and simmer, covered, until the potatoes break apart when stirred, about 15 minutes. Potatoes will become very sticky. If they start to stick to the bottom of the saucepan, remove it from the heat, stir, and return to the heat.

2. Place potatoes in a blender or food processor and blend until very smooth and creamy, about 5 minutes.

3. Return them to the saucepan and add all other ingredients. Simmer, covered, for 10 minutes.

GAZPACHO

Makes 10 cups

Make this wonderful cold Spanish soup ahead—it takes 12 to 24 hours in the refrigerator to be just right.

1 28-oz. can tomatoes, chopped, or 3½ C chopped fresh tomatoes

1 cucumber, peeled and diced

1 medium onion, chopped

1 green pepper, seeded and chopped

4½ C water

¼ tsp. garlic powder

3 tsp. olive oil

2 T vinegar

salt and pepper to taste.

Place the tomatoes in a large mixing bowl and mash. Add all other ingredients and mix thoroughly. Cover and refrigerate for 12 to 24 hours before serving.

LENTIL PARSNIP SOUP

Serves six to eight

6 C water

1 C lentils

3 T natural soy sauce

⅛ tsp. pepper

1 bay leaf

1 tsp. cold-pressed olive oil

½ onion, chopped

1 leek, sliced

1 clove garlic, chopped

1 celery stalk

1 parsnip, diced

2 carrots, diced

2 T chopped parsley

dash of ground cloves

1. In a large soup pot place the water, lentils, soy sauce, pepper, and bay leaf. Bring to a boil and cook for 1½ hours.

2. In the meantime, heat the oil in a large skillet. Sauté the onions until golden brown. Add the leek, garlic, celery, parsnip, carrots, parsley, and cloves. Mix well, cover, and cook for 5 minutes.

3. Add the skillet mixture to the lentils and cook for 30 minutes. Add ½ to 1 cup of boiling water to the soup if it becomes too thick.

NOTE. Remove the bay leaf before serving.

MIXED LEGUME SOUP

Serves six

¼ C navy beans, soaked overnight

¼ C baby lima beans, soaked overnight

¼ C split peas

¼ C pearl barley

2 qt. water or vegetable stock

1 tsp. salt

1 onion, chopped

1 clove garlic, chopped

2 large carrots, sliced

1 celery stalk, sliced

1 leek, light end only, sliced

2 T nutritional yeast

⅛ tsp. pepper

½ tsp. onion powder

½ tsp. garlic powder

¼ tsp. thyme

⅛ tsp. ground cloves

½ bay leaf

¼ tsp. ground celery seeds

1. Place the navy beans, lima beans, split peas, pearl barley, and water in a large soup pot. Add the salt, bring to a boil, and cook for 40 minutes.

2. Add the rest of the ingredients and cook for 30 minutes more. Adjust the seasoning and serve with fresh whole wheat bread and a large green salad.

LENTIL SOUP WITH FRESH CILANTRO

Serves eight

In the high desert beyond Los Angeles is a small Benedictine monastery, where the monks run a guesthouse. Carmin, who prepares food for monks and guests alike, makes this tasty and easy-to-prepare soup. The long cooking time makes it creamy.

11 C water

2 C lentils, washed and cleaned

1 tsp. salt

1 onion, finely chopped

¼ tsp. ground cumin seed

⅛ tsp. pepper

2 tomatoes, diced

1 T coarsely chopped cilantro

1. Bring the water to a boil in a large pot. Add the lentils, salt, onion, cumin, and pepper. Simmer, covered, for 2½ hours.

2. Add the tomatoes and cook, covered, for 30 minutes. Add the cilantro and cook for 15 minutes. Serve with warm tortillas and fresh steamed corn on the cob.

POTATO, TOMATO, AND
CARROT SOUP WITH BASIL

Serves six

While this soup might sound plain, it's really very elegant and very pretty.

6 *medium potatoes, peeled*
water
1 *C fresh or canned*
tomatoes, with liquid,
cut into chunks
2 *carrots, cut into match*
sticks

1 *T chopped fresh basil*
1 *C Mushroom Stock (page*
109)
salt and pepper to taste
6 *small sprigs parsley to*
garnish

1. Dice the potatoes. Place in a saucepan with water to cover. Cook until just tender.

2. Place two-thirds of the potatoes in a blender or food processor and blend until very smooth. Return all the potatoes to the saucepan and add the rest of the ingredients. Bring to a boil and simmer, covered, until the carrots are just tender. Garnish each bowl of soup with a sprig of parsley.

VICHYSSOISE

Serves eight

2 tsp. cold-pressed olive oil

4 medium leeks, whites only, washed well and thinly sliced

1 medium onion, chopped

4 medium potatoes, thinly sliced

3 C vegetable stock or prepared instant broth

¼ tsp. tarragon

½ tsp. salt

⅛ tsp. white pepper

2 C mild soy milk

2 T chopped chives

sliced cucumber (2 or 3 slices per bowl)

1. Heat the oil in a large saucepan, add the leeks and onion, and cook until golden. Do not allow the onion to burn or the taste will be bitter and there will be dark specks in this creamy white soup.

2. Add the potatoes, stock, tarragon, salt, and pepper. Cover and bring to a boil. Reduce heat and cook about 30 minutes or until the potatoes are tender. If the liquid is absorbed before the cooking is complete, add a little water.

3. Pass through a sieve or cream in a food processsor until smooth. Stir in the soy milk and adjust seasonings. Serve the soup hot in individual bowls or serve it cold in individual bowls by chilling for 2 hours. When ready to serve, sprinkle chopped chives on top and garnish with slices of cold cucumber.

MANHATTAN CHOWDER

Serves 6

No clams, of course, but what a taste!

1 *tsp. cold-pressed olive oil*

1 *large onion, chopped*

2 *carrots, diced*

1 *celery stalk, sliced*

10 *sprigs parsley, chopped*

28 *oz. cooked* or *canned tomatoes, crushed*

5 *C water*

1 *tsp. salt*

¼ *tsp. ground black pepper*

⅛ *tsp. white pepper*

1 *bay leaf*

1 *tsp. ground thyme*

3 *medium potatoes, diced*

2 *T nutritional yeast (omit for yeast-free diets)*

2 *T dry wakami sea vegetable, crumbled (optional)*

soup crackers

1. Heat the oil in a large saucepan. Add the onion, carrots, and celery and cook until the onion is transparent, about 7 minutes. Add the parsley, tomatoes, water, salt, pepper, bay leaf, and thyme. Bring to a boil, reduce heat, and simmer for 40 minutes.

2. Add the potatoes, nutritional yeast, and wakami and cook for 20 minutes more or until the potatoes are tender but not mushy. Wakami adds a seafood flavor. Crumble the soup crackers into the chowder and serve hot.

NOTE. Remove the bay leaf before serving.

MULLIGATAWNY

Serves six

This soup is rich and has an East Indian flavor.

¾ C water

¼ C grated dried coconut

2 tsp. cold-pressed vegetable oil

1 onion, chopped

1 carrot, sliced

1 celery stalk, sliced

2 green apples, cored and chopped

½ C garbanzo beans, soaked overnight (Sprouted garbanzo may be used without soaking.)

2 tsp. curry powder

1 tsp. salt

⅓ tsp. pepper

¼ tsp. thyme

1 bay leaf

2 T chopped fresh parsley

½ tsp. lemon rind

1 tsp. fresh, grated ginger

4 C water

8 small new potatoes

1 C cooked brown rice

1. Boil ¾ cup of water and the coconut for 1 minute and let it stand for 1 hour. Place it in a blender at high speed for 3 minutes. Strain through a clean, damp, gauze diaper or a double layer of damp cheesecloth. Wring the pulp to extract as much liquid as possible. Refrigerate the milk and discard the pulp. Two-thirds of a cup of natural, unsweetened coconut milk (not the clear liquid found in a fresh green coconut) may be used in place of the homemade coconut milk.

2. Heat the oil in a skillet and cook the onion, carrot, celery, and apples for 5 minutes, covered. Do not allow the onion to brown.

3. Place the garbanzo beans in a blender or food processor and grind to the texture of coarse corn meal.

4. Add the ground garbanzos, curry, salt, pepper, and thyme to the cooking vegetables and cook for 3 minutes. Transfer the skillet mixture to a saucepan and add the bay leaf, parsley, lemon rind, ginger, and 4 cups of water and cook for 50 minutes.

5. Meanwhile, steam the new potatoes until they are tender. Cool

them for 5 minutes, slip off the skins, and cut them in halves or fourths. Set them aside.

6. Strain the vegetable mixture or purée in a blender. Return the soup to the saucepan, add the rice, and cook for 10 minutes. Add the pota-toes and cook for 5 minutes. Turn off the heat and stir in the coconut milk. When reheating, do not boil.

NOTE: Remove the bay leaf before serving.

FAST VEGETABLE CREAM SOUP

Serves four

The chefs at Arrowhead Mills came up with this very quick and easy-to-make soup. It's perfect for those evenings when you really don't feel like cooking but want to serve something satisfying.

> 2 C fresh vegetables (such as peas, broccoli, corn, cauliflower, carrots, or zucchini)
>
> ½ C sesame tahini
>
> 2 C water
>
> 4 T white miso or 4 tsp. soy sauce

Place all the ingredients in a blender or food processor and blend until creamy. Bring to a boil and cook for 3 minutes.

GUMBO

Serves six

1 *tsp. cold-pressed olive oil*

¼ *onion, chopped*

1 *clove garlic, finely chopped*

2 *C fresh or canned tomatoes, chopped, liquid included*

¼ *lb. okra, sliced*

¼ *lb. fresh lemon, sliced*

¼ *green pepper, chopped*

corn kernels from 1 ear

3 *C water*

1 *bay leaf*

½ *tsp. salt*

¼ *tsp. paprika*

dash cayenne

2 *tsp. natural soy sauce*

2 *T whole wheat pastry flour*

4 *T water*

1 *tsp. vinegar*

1. Heat the oil in a soup pot. Add the onion and cook until transparent. Stir in the garlic and cook for 1 minute. Add the tomatoes, okra, lemon, pepper, and corn and cook, covered, for 5 minutes. Add the 3 cups of water, bay leaf, salt, paprika, cayenne, and soy sauce and simmer for 1 hour.

2. Mix the flour into the 4 tablespoons of water and the vinegar. Slowly add this mixture to the soup, stirring briskly until completely mixed. Continue stirring until the soup has thickened and then serve.

SPLIT PEA SOUP

Serves eight

1 *lb. dry green split peas*

1 *tsp. mild cold-pressed olive oil*

1 *clove garlic, chopped*

1 *leek, chopped*

½ *onion, chopped*

1 *celery stalk, chopped*

1 *carrot, chopped*

⅛ *tsp. pepper*

½ *bay leaf*

1 *tsp. salt*

dash of thyme

1. Clean the split peas and let them stand overnight in 2½ quarts of water. Or clean the split peas, boil in 2½ quarts of water for 2 minutes, and let them stand for 1 hour.

2. Heat the olive oil in a large skillet. Add the garlic, leek, onion, celery, and carrot, and sauté over medium heat for 10 minutes.

3. Add the sautéed vegetables and all the other ingredients to the split peas, bring to a boil, and simmer for 2 hours. As foam appears, skim it off and discard. Serve the soup with whole wheat Croutons (page 119).

YAM AND SPLIT PEA SOUP WITH FRESH GINGER

Serves eight

2 C dried split peas

3 medium yams, peeled and
    diced

3 leeks, diced

2 T diced fresh ginger

4 celery stalks, diced

3 carrots, diced

1 tsp. salt

3 T Braggs Aminos

water

⅛ tsp. cayenne pepper

Place all the ingredients except the cayenne pepper in a large pot. Add water so that there are 2 inches of water over the vegetables. Cover, bring to a boil, turn down heat, and simmer for 2 hours, or until all the ingredients are mushy. Stir often to prevent sticking. If the soup becomes too thick while it is cooking, add some boiling water, or you can thin it with a bit of water at the end of the cooking time for a lighter soup. Add cayenne pepper, adjust the seasonings, and serve.

ORIENTAL SOUP

Serves four

6 *C water*

2 *scallions, thinly sliced*

4 *thin slices fresh ginger*

6 *mushrooms, sliced*

8 *snow peas, strings removed*

2 *T dry sherry*

2 *T soy sauce*

dash pepper

2 *T light miso*

1. Bring the water to a boil. Add the scallions and ginger and simmer, covered, for 20 minutes.

2. Add the mushrooms, snow peas, dry sherry, soy sauce, and pepper to this broth and cook 10 minutes more. Remove from the heat. Dissolve the miso in 2 tablespoons of the soup broth and stir it into the soup. Serve at once.

CAULIFLOWER SOUP

Serves four

This soup is creamy white and rich, elegant enough for a dinner party.

1 *tsp. cold-pressed olive oil*

1 *onion, chopped*

3 *garlic cloves, thinly sliced*

4 *C vegetable stock* or *broth*

1 *cauliflower, broken into florets, stem diced*

1 *C mild soy milk*

⅛ *tsp. pepper*

salt to taste

1 *T chopped parsley* or *chives to garnish*

croutons (optional)

1. Heat the oil in a large skillet. Add the onion and cook slowly for about 10 minutes until they are translucent. Do not allow the onions to brown. Turn up the heat just a little, add the garlic, and cook for 1 minute. Add the stock, cauliflower, soy milk, pepper, and salt and simmer, covered, for 45 minutes.

2. Put three-fourths of the soup into a blender and purée until very creamy. Return the creamed soup to the skillet. Heat before serving. Garnish with a sprinkling of chopped parsley or chopped chives. Some croutons added to each bowl when serving gives a pleasant crunch.

MUSHROOM STOCK

Makes 8 cups

The hearty taste of this stock comes from aged mushrooms, that is, fresh mushrooms that have been stored in a paper bag in the refrigerator for at least a week.

1 *large onion, chopped*
1 *T cold-pressed olive oil*
½ *lb. aged mushrooms*

8 *C water*
1 *carrot*

1. Sauté the onion in olive oil at medium-high heat for seven minutes, or until golden. Stir constantly so that the onion does not burn.

2. Combine the onions with the other ingredients in a large saucepan or stock pot and simmer for 1 hour. Strain through a sieve and discard the onions and mushrooms.

VEGETABLE STOCK

The easiest of all stocks to make is the byproduct of your regular cooking. When you steam or boil vegetables, don't throw out the water. Pour it into a plastic container, store in the refrigerator, and just keep adding to it. After several days close it and freeze for later use. Do not use a glass jar. It could explode in the process of freezing as the contents expand. Use water from cooked onions, green beans, peas, potatoes, carrots, spinach, squash, parsnip, or any other mild-flavored vegetables. But to make a rich vegetable stock, just follow the recipe below.

2 *onions, chopped*
4 *carrots, chopped*
3 *celery stalks, chopped*
1 *clove garlic, chopped*
½ *C week-old mushrooms, chopped*

Peels and parings from tomatoes, peppers, potatoes, carrots, and other such vegetables
water

Place all the ingredients in a pot. Cover with water and simmer, covered, for about 1 hour or more. Strain out the vegetables and discard them. The broth will be very bland. Season to taste and cook for 15 minutes more.

NOTE. Don't use cabbage, broccoli, cauliflower, brussels sprouts, or turnip parings since they have a very strong taste, which could overwhelm the flavor of the stock.

9

SALADS, DRESSINGS, AND CONDIMENTS

MIDDLE EASTERN SALAD

Serves six

Serve this fresh-tasting salad as a filling for pita sandwiches, as a chutney to cool off spicy dishes such as curries, or as a salad.

4 *large ripe tomatoes, cut into bite-size chunks*

1 *cucumber, peeled and sliced (if you are using a hot-house cucumber do not peel)*

1 *C coarsely chopped parsley*

4 *medium fresh basil leaves, chopped*

Sesame Tahini Dressing *(page 132)*

Toss tomatoes, cucumber, parsley, and basil together. Add dressing to taste.

MIXED GREENS SALAD
WITH FRESH DILL

Serves six

The best-tasting and most nutritious salads contain a variety of lettuces and greens with some other raw vegetables thrown in for color and texture. Some tasty greens to try are watercress, spinach, kale, chard, mustard greens, parsley, beet greens, celery tops, and green cabbage. Raw vegetables such as tomatoes, jicama, and cucumbers add interest.

1 *head green leaf lettuce*
1 *bunch watercress*
½ *bunch fresh parsley*
4 *T fresh dill, leaves only, chopped*
1 *tomato, sliced into wedges*
½ *cucumber, peeled and thinly sliced or ¼ hot-house cucumber, unpeeled and thinly sliced*
2 *T cold-pressed mild olive oil*
juice of ½ lemon
¼ *tsp. salt*
⅛ *tsp. pepper*

1. Wash and dry the lettuce and break it into bite-size pieces. Wash the watercress several times, dry, remove the stems, and cut the leaves into bite-size pieces. Wash and dry the parsley, remove the leaves, and discard the stems.

2. Combine the lettuce, watercress, parsley, dill, tomato, and cucumber in a large salad bowl. Combine the olive oil and lemon and sprinkle over the salad. Season with salt and pepper and toss well. Serve immediately.

SALADE NIÇOISE

Serves four

This salad is a traditional one from the south of France. Usually it includes cooked fish and hard-boiled eggs, but our version is just as tasty and fun to eat.

1 *clove garlic*

2 *T cold-pressed olive oil*

6 *new potatoes*

1 *T natural soy sauce*

1 *T white wine vinegar*

10 *green beans, ends and strings removed*

1 *head Boston lettuce*

¼ *tsp. salt*

⅛ *tsp. pepper*

1 *T fresh lemon juice*

1 *tsp. Dijon-style mustard*

1 *tsp. tomato paste*

1 *T white wine*

8 *Greek olives*

2 *medium tomatoes, cut into 12 wedges each*

1. Slice the clove of garlic and soak it in the olive oil for about 30 minutes, then discard the garlic and reserve the oil.

2. Steam the potatoes until they are just tender when pricked with a fork. The skins should not split. Soak the cooked potatoes in cold water for 1 minute. They will still be warm but cool enough to handle. Slip off the skins and slice into moderately thin pieces. Combine the soy sauce and vinegar in a bowl, add the sliced potatoes, and toss. Cover and let stand until the rest of the salad is prepared.

3. Break the green beans into thirds and steam for 4 minutes or until barely tender. Set aside to cool.

4. Wash and dry the lettuce and break it into bite-size pieces. In the bottom of a large salad bowl combine the salt, pepper, lemon juice, mustard, tomato paste, wine, and garlic oil. Whisk well until emulsified. Add the lettuce, potatoes, and their juice, if any, and the green beans and olives. Toss well. Garnish with the tomato wedges and serve immediately.

CHILEAN SALAD

Serves six

Chilean geographer Carlos Hagen-Lautrup is director of the UCLA map library and an expert chef, among other things. This adaptation of the popular Chilean summer salad is one of his favorites.

2 *large red onions (preferably a sweet variety)*

2 *T salt*

6 *C cold water*

7 *large ripe tomatoes, cut into bite-size chunks*

½ *C (1 bunch) finely chopped cilantro*

½ *C (1 bunch) finely chopped parsley*

⅓ *C cold-pressed olive oil*

½ *C fresh lemon juice*

½ *tsp. pepper*

1. Thinly slice the onions so that each slice is nearly translucent. In a large bowl mix the salt and water. Add the onions and marinate in the refrigerator for 4 to 5 hours. Discard the soaking liquid and rinse the onions in cold water. Let them drain for a couple of minutes in a colander.

2. Combine the marinated onions with the remaining ingredients and toss well. Add more lemon juice and pepper if desired. Serve immediately. This salad loses its crispness and fresh taste when refrigerated for more than 1 or 2 hours. Chilean salad is a pleasant "mouth cooler" when served with a curry dish or a spicy falafel.

VARIATION. Add chile powder or finely chopped garlic for a spicier version.

TABBOULEH SALAD

Serves six

Carlos Hagen-Lautrup is as fond of Mediterranean cooking as he is of his native Chilean foods. We chose this recipe from his collection because of its versatility and popularity.

1 C bulgur (precooked cracked wheat)

water

½ C chopped green onions

4 medium tomatoes, diced

juice of one large lemon

1 bunch parsley, finely chopped

1 small bunch mint, finely chopped (about ⅓ C)

1 tsp. salt

½ tsp. freshly ground pepper

¼ C cold-pressed olive oil

Romaine lettuce leaves, washed and dried

1. Soak the bulgur in just enough water to cover. If you add a little too much water, drain it off immediately. Soaking times vary according to your taste. For a chewy texture soak for about 30 minutes; for a soft texture soak for up to 2 hours.

2. In the meantime, prepare the other ingredients. Mix the onions, tomatoes, lemon juice, parsley, mint, salt, pepper, and oil in a salad bowl. Add the soaked bulgur and mix well. Serve on a bed of romaine lettuce. Feel free to vary the amounts of any of the ingredients, according to your taste, or even to add your own. This salad will keep, refrigerated, for up to 5 days.

CHINESE GREEN SALAD

Serves four to six

This salad is the perfect companion to any Oriental-style meal. As with any green salad, dressing should be added at the last minute before serving.

6 *Napa cabbage leaves,*
   large

1 *medium head green leaf*
   lettuce

¼ *hot-house cucumber (or ⅓*
   regular cucumber)

2 *oz. Chinese pea pods,*
   stems and strings
   removed

¼ *C bean sprouts*

Ginger Tamari Dressing
   (page 131)

5 *whole wheat sesame*
   crackers, broken into
   bite-size pieces

1. Wash and dry the cabbage. Slice the leaves into ½-inch-wide pieces and cut the stalks into slices ⅕ inch thick.

2. Wash and dry the lettuce and tear into bite-size pieces.

3. Cut the washed, unpeeled cucumber into thin slices. If a regular cucumber is used, peel first.

4. Mix the cabbage, lettuce, cucumber, pea pods, and bean sprouts in a large salad bowl. Cover with ¼ cup of the dressing and toss. Taste and add more dressing if desired. Serve with crackers.

Romaine, Carrot, and Walnut Salad with Cranberry Dressing

Serves four to six

2 *heads romaine lettuce*

3 *carrots, peeled*

¾ *C Hawthorne Cranberry Dressing (page 132)*

½ *C chopped walnuts*

4 to 6 *walnut halves*

1. Wash the lettuce, then dry and break into bite-size pieces.

2. Cut the carrots into matchstick pieces about 1½ inches long and ⅛ inch thick.

3. Pour ½ cup of the dressing over the lettuce and chopped walnuts in a large salad bowl and toss lightly. Toss the carrots in a separate bowl with the remaining dressing.

4. Place the carrots in the center of the romaine and garnish with walnut halves.

Spinach and Mushroom Salad with Cucumber Dressing

Serves four

1 *clove garlic, sliced*

4 *T cold-pressed olive oil*

2 *bunches spinach*

6 *medium mushrooms, sliced*

2 *T white wine vinegar*

1 *T natural soy sauce*

1½ *to 2 inches of cucumber, sliced*

½ *tsp. salt*

⅛ *tsp. pepper*

½ *C Croutons (page 119)*

1. Soak the garlic in the olive oil for 30 minutes.

2. Cut off the stems of the spinach and save for soup stock. Wash the leaves well several times, then dry. Place the spinach leaves and mushrooms in a large salad bowl.

3. Remove the garlic from the oil and discard the garlic. In a blender, combine the olive oil, vinegar, soy sauce, cucumber, salt, and pepper and blend until creamy. Pour over the spinach and mushrooms and toss until coated. Sprinkle croutons on top and serve immediately.

CAESAR SALAD

Serves four

1 *clove garlic, sliced*
3 *T cold-pressed olive oil*
½ *tsp. dry mustard*
1 *T lemon juice*
1 *T white wine vinegar*
2 *tsp. natural soy sauce*

6 *Greek olives, pitted and*
   chopped into a paste
2 *bunches romaine lettuce,*
   washed, dried, and torn
   into bite-size pieces
1 *C Croutons (page 119)*

1. Soak the garlic in the olive oil for 30 minutes, then remove the garlic and discard.

2. In a jar, combine the olive oil, mustard, lemon juice, vinegar, soy sauce, and Greek olive paste. Secure lid and shake until the dressing is emulsified.

3. Place the lettuce in a large salad bowl and toss with the dressing. Sprinkle with croutons and serve immediately.

CROUTONS

Makes about 3 cups

2 *tsp. vinegar*
2 *tsp. water*
3 *slices whole wheat bread*

salt
garlic powder

1. Preheat the oven to 250°F. Mix the vinegar and water and brush each slice of bread lightly with this mixture. Place on a baking sheet, sprinkle with salt and garlic, and bake for 30 minutes.

2. Remove from the oven, cut into ½-inch cubes, and return to the oven for 15 to 30 minutes more or until the croutons are crisp. Do not allow to darken or the croutons will be bitter. Cool.

3. When completely cooled, store in a closed container or plastic bag.

VARIATIONS. For an Italian flavor, sprinkle with basil before baking. For a Mexican flavor, sprinkle with chile powder. For Borscht (page 91), make the croutons out of rye bread.

TACO SALAD

Serves six

¼ *green pepper, very finely chopped*

1 *green onion, finely chopped*

2 *T finely chopped cilantro*

3 *T cold-pressed olive oil, or 1 T cold-pressed olive oil and 2 T Eden Oil Substitute (page 133)*

1 *T white vinegar*

1 *T fresh lemon juice*

¼ *tsp. salt*

¼ *tsp. chile powder*

1 *clove garlic, bruised with a fork*

1 *head green leaf lettuce, washed and broken into bite-size pieces*

¼ *C sliced black olives*

1 *tomato, diced*

½ *C broken tortilla chips or corn chips*

½ *C Guacamole (page 55)*

6 *whole black olives*

1. Make the dressing in a small bowl by mixing the green pepper, green onion, cilantro, olive oil, vinegar, lemon juice, salt, chile powder, and bruised garlic clove. Whisk and allow to stand for 30 minutes. Remove the garlic clove and discard.

2. In a large salad bowl mix the lettuce, sliced olives, tomato, and tortilla chips. Cover with the dressing and toss.

3. Serve on large salad dishes with a generous dab of guacamole on top. Garnish with a whole black olive.

RED CABBAGE AND MUSTARD GREEN SALAD

Serves six

The vivid violet of the cabbage against the bright green of the mustard greens makes this salad truly beautiful. Garnish it with a small purple orchid and watch your table light up.

1 *small head red cabbage*
8 *large mustard leaves*

1 *C Ginger Tamari*
Dressing (omit the
sesame seeds) (page 131)

1. Remove the dark or wilted outer cabbage leaves. Cut into quarters and slice thinly.

2. Wash and dry the mustard greens. Remove the stems and cut the leaves into pieces about ¼ inch wide.

3. Combine the cabbage, mustard greens, and dressing in a salad bowl and toss well.

CARROT ALMOND SALAD

Serves six

8 *carrots, grated and chilled*
½ *C sliced almonds*

Ginger Vinaigrette (page 130)

Toss the carrots and almonds with the dressing and serve immediately.

COLESLAW

Serves eight

1 *head red cabbage,*
   shredded

2 *apples, grated*

2 *carrots, grated*

4 *green onions, finely*
   chopped

2 *T vinegar*

½ *tsp. salt*

½ *tsp. pepper*

1 *tsp. soy sauce*

4 *T Mayo Spread I or II*
   (pages 87, 88) or
   mayonnaise

1 *tsp. crushed caraway*
   seeds

Mix together all the ingredients and refrigerate, covered, for 4 to 12 hours.

FRENCH POTATO SALAD

Serves four

3 *large white potatoes*

1 *green onion, finely sliced*

1 *T soy sauce*

2 *tsp. vinegar*

2 *tsp. water*

¼ *tsp. ground black pepper*

1 *T cold-pressed vegetable*
   oil

3 *T Mayo Spread I or II*
   (pages 87, 88) or
   mayonnaise

1. Steam the potatoes in their skins until just tender. Do not allow the skins to split. Soak in cold water for 5 minutes until cool enough to handle but still warm.

2. Slip off the skins, cut into slices, and set aside.

3. In a bowl large enough to hold the finished potato salad, mix the

onion, soy sauce, vinegar, water, and pepper. Slowly add the oil, whisking constantly. Add the Mayo Spread and mix well.

4. While the potatoes are still warm, add them to the dressing and toss gently with a wooden spoon. Refrigerate for at least 1 hour before serving.

POTATO SALAD WITH DILL SAUCE

Serves four to six

Creamy white potatoes studded with pale green and pink in a delicate dill sauce makes this salad perfect for luncheons.

10 *new red potatoes*
2 *large celery stalks with greens, sliced*
1 *T chopped pimentos*
1 *T chopped parsley*

1 *T cold-pressed mild olive oil*
1 *T fresh lemon juice*
¼ *C Dill Sauce (page 136)*

1. Wash the potatoes and steam them until just tender. Do not allow the skins to split. Soak the cooked potatoes in ice water for 5 minutes then cut the potatoes into slices ¼ inch thick.

2. Mix together the remaining ingredients, combine with the potatoes, and toss gently until all the potatoes are coated.

Cold Asparagus Salad

Serves four

2 lb. fresh asparagus

½ cup Mayo Spread I or II (pages 87, 88) or mayonnaise

1 T cold-pressed olive oil

1 T lemon juice

1 tsp. Dijon mustard

1. Wash the asparagus. Trim away the tough ends and peel the last 2 or 3 inches if necessary. Place about 2 inches of water in a covered roasting pan that is long enough to accommodate the length of the asparagus. Salt the water and bring to a boil. Add the asparagus and cook, covered, until tender, about 13 minutes. Drain and refrigerate, covered, for ½ hour.

2. In a small bowl whisk together the remaining ingredients and refrigerate. When the asparagus is chilled pour the dressing over and serve.

Garbanzo Bean Salad

Serves six to eight

2 T cold-pressed olive oil, or 1 T cold-pressed olive oil and 1 T Eden Oil Substitute (page 133)

1 T white vinegar

salt and pepper to taste

¼ tsp. garlic powder

4 C cooked garbanzo beans

1 T pimentos or roasted peppers, chopped (Canned pimentos may be used.)

1 green onion, finely chopped

Combine the oil, vinegar, salt, pepper, and garlic powder in a small salad bowl and whisk. Add the beans, pimentos, and green onion and toss well. Chill before serving.

LEFTOVER VEGETABLE SALAD

Serves six

Last night's crisp steamed veggies become today's perky vegetable salad. The purpose of this suggestion is to stimulate your imagination.

2 C steamed vegetables (whatever you happen to have)

1 scallion, includiong greens, chopped

½ sweet red pepper, thinly sliced

3 T of your favorite salad dressing or Mayo Spread I or II (pages 87, 88)

Fresh ground pepper

Combine all the ingredients and toss well.

AVOCADO AND JICAMA SALAD

Serves six

Nothing can match the creamy richness of ripe avocados, or the surprising sweet crunch of jicama.

2 ripe (not darkened) avocados

1 C jicama, peeled, quartered, and sliced

½ C French Vinaigrette (page 130)

6 large lettuce leaves, washed and dried

1. Cut the avocados in half around the pit. Twist to separate the halves, then remove the pit and peel. Cut lengthwise into slices.

2. In a salad bowl mix the avocado, jicama, and vinaigrette and toss gently until completely coated. Chill.

3. Place a lettuce leaf on six individual salad plates and serve the salad.

AVOCADO STUFFED WITH WATER CHESTNUTS AND WALNUTS

Serves four

2 *large ripe avocados*

4 *large lettuce leaves, washed and dried*

½ *C Mayo Spread I or II (pages 87, 88) or mayonnaise*

1 *tsp. tomato paste*

dash pepper

1 *tsp. chopped capers*

1½ *C (12 oz.) sliced water chestnuts*

2 *small celery stalks, thinly sliced (use the light, tender stalks in the center of the bunch)*

½ *C walnuts, broken*

¼ *C sliced black olives*

4 *tomato wedges*

4 *whole black olives*

1. Cut the avocados into halves and remove the pits. Carefully peel, keeping each half intact. Place a lettuce leaf on a salad dish and place each avocado half, cut side up, on the lettuce leaf.

2. In a mixing bowl whisk together the Mayo Spread or mayonnaise, tomato paste, pepper, and capers. Add the water chestnuts, celery, walnuts, and black olives and toss until well mixed.

3. Place one quarter of the water chestnut mixture in the center of each avocado. Garnish with a tomato wedge and an olive.

AVOCADO, TOMATO, AND CUCUMBER SALAD

Refreshing, bright, and tasty.

1 *ripe firm avocado*

1 *large ripe tomato, washed*

½ *cucumber, peeled* or ¼ *hot-house cucumber, unpeeled*

¼ *C French Vinaigrette (page 130)*

1. Cut the avocado in half, then remove the pit and skin. Cut, widthwise, into slices.

2. Cut the tomato into quarters, then into slices.

3. Cut the cucumber into ⅛-inch slices.

4. Combine in a mixing bowl the vegetables and the vinaigrette and toss just enough to coat the vegetables completely. Serve immediately.

CALIFORNIA WINTER
FRUIT SALAD

Serves two

This dish is rich and creamy and makes a perfect, healthful breakfast or a light dessert.

1 *ripe pear*

1 *apple*

1 *peeled banana*

1 *T walnut pieces*

1 *T raw, unsalted sunflower seeds*

½ *T Almond Butter (page 90) or Cashew Butter (page 89)*

1 *T natural maple syrup*

1. Core and cut the pear and apple into bite-size pieces. Slice half of the banana. Mix the pear, apple, banana slices, walnuts, and sunflower seeds in a bowl.

2. In a separate bowl, mash the other half of the banana and mix in the almond butter and maple syrup.

3. Spoon over fruit and mix well until all the pieces are coated.

AMBROSIA SALAD

Serves four

As the first course of a summer supper or as dessert for lunch or dinner, this salad is as pretty as it is delicious.

3 oranges, peeled

3 bananas (ripe but not brown)

juice of 1 orange

1 T shredded coconut

1 T date sugar (ground dried dates)

3 strawberries or 3 slices kiwi fruit for garnish

Sprig of mint for garnish

1. Separate the oranges into sections. With a sharp knife cut away the white pith on the bottom rounded part of each wedge. Peel the bananas and cut into slices ⅛ to ¼ inch thick and toss in 2 tablespoons of orange juice. In a separate bowl, combine the coconut and date sugar.

2. Moisten the bottom of a pretty, not too large, serving bowl with a tablespoon of orange juice. Lay a single layer of bananas on the bottom and sprinkle with a bit of the coconut–date-sugar mixture. Arrange the orange slices in a pinwheel design over the bananas. Sprinkle with more orange juice and coconut/date sugar. Continue with another layer of bananas, coconut/date sugar, oranges, and so on, until all the fruit is used up. Garnish with strawberries or kiwi fruit in the middle of the pinwheel and a sprig of mint on the side.

FRENCH VINAIGRETTE

Makes 1 cup

This sauce is just about the most versatile one there is. It makes a delicious dressing for green salads and three-bean salad, it is a dip for artichokes and asparagus, and it is a marinade for Jerusalem artichokes.

1 *garlic clove, sliced*
5 T *cold-pressed olive oil, or* 2 T *olive oil and 3 T Eden Oil Substitute (page 133)*

1 *tsp. honey*
2 *tsp. hot water*
4 T *white vinegar*
¼ *tsp. ground black pepper*
¼ *tsp. salt*

Place the garlic in the olive oil and let stand ½ hour. Remove the garlic and discard. Combine the olive oil with the remaining ingredients and whisk lightly. This keeps for about 2 weeks.

NOTE. Half of the oil can be replaced with the Oil Substitute to cut fat. For severely fat-restricted diets, replace all oil with Oil Substitute.

GINGER VINAIGRETTE

Makes ⅔ cup

2 *tsp. honey*
1 T *vinegar*
1 T *fresh lemon juice*
1 T *fresh grated ginger*

⅓ *tsp. salt*
4 T *cold-pressed olive oil, or* 2 T *cold-pressed olive oil and 2 T Eden Oil Substitute (page 133)*

1. Dissolve the honey in the vinegar and lemon juice.

2. Add the remaining ingredients, mix well, and chill.

3. Serve over Carrot Almond Salad (page 121), sliced cucumbers, avocado, asparagus, or mixed greens. This keeps for 3 days.

RUSSIAN DRESSING

Makes 1¼ cups

1 C Mayo Spread (page 87)
    or *mayonnaise*

1½ T prepared horseradish
    or 1 T fresh grated
    horseradish

1 tsp. grated onion

2 T tomato paste

Place all the ingredients in a blender
and purée. This keeps for 1 week.

GINGER TAMARI DRESSING

Makes 1 cup

1 T finely grated fresh
    ginger

1 tsp. honey

1 T natural tamari soy
    sauce

1 T white wine vinegar
    (preferably rice vinegar)

2 T fresh lemon juice

¼ C cold-pressed olive oil,
    or 2 T cold-pressed
    olive oil and 2 T Eden
    Oil Substitute (page 133)

1 T raw hulled sesame seeds

1. Put the ginger, honey, tamari,
and vinegar in a small bowl. Let the
mixture stand for 5 minutes, then
whisk to blend.

2. Add the remaining ingredients
and whisk again. Refrigerate. This
keeps for 3 days.

SESAME TAHINI DRESSING

Makes 1⅔ cups

¾ C tahini

1½ T Braggs Aminos or
natural mild soy sauce

4½ T water

juice of 1 lemon

Mix all the ingredients until emulsified. Serve over Middle Eastern Salad (page 111), sliced tomatoes, or sliced cucumbers.

HAWTHORNE CRANBERRY DRESSING

Makes ⅔ cup

Across the street from the Witches' Museum, in Salem, Massachusetts, is a charming hotel called the Hawthorne Hotel. This exciting salad dressing is served in their dining room.

¼ C red wine

2 T finely sliced cranberries

2 tsp. chopped green onions

2 tsp. honey

¼ C cold-pressed vegetable
oil, or 2 T cold-pressed
olive oil and 2 T Eden
Oil Substitute (page 133)

1. Mix together the wine, cranberries, green onions, and honey.

2. Slowly add the oil (or oil substitute, if you are using it), whisking all the while.

EDEN OIL SUBSTITUTE

Makes 1⅔ cups

This recipe comes to us from Eden Foods. Replace all or part of the oil in any cold salad dressing with this oil substitute.

⅓ C water

½ T agar flakes

1 C mild soy milk

1. Place the water and agar in a small saucepan and simmer, stirring often, until the agar is dissolved, 5 to 8 minutes.

2. Pour the soy milk into a blender and add the agar mixture. Add all the other ingredients, blend until smooth, and chill for 45 minutes. If making it to have on hand, store it in a closed container in the refrigerator without adding the other dressing ingredients, and use in place of oil in salad dressings.

POPPY SEED DRESSING

Makes 2 cups

1⅔ C Eden Oil Substitute (page 133)

2 T toasted sesame oil

1 T brown rice vinegar or red wine vinegar

1 clove garlic, pressed

1 tsp. sea salt

2 tsp. poppy seeds

1. Place all the ingredients in a blender and blend until smooth. Chill 45 minutes and blend again.

2. Store the dressing in a closed container for up to 10 days.

CREAMY OIL SUBSTITUTE

Makes 1⅔ cups

By substituting this for part or all of the oil in a recipe, you can convert any salad dressing into a creamy dressing with less fat.

⅔ C water

½ tsp. agar flakes

1 tsp. arrowroot

1 C mild soy milk

1. Place the water and agar in a small saucepan and simmer, stirring often, until the agar is completely dissolved, 5 to 8 minutes.

2. Dissolve the arrowroot in one tablespoon of the soy milk and add to the agar mixture, whisking briskly. Boil and cook for 2 minutes more, stirring constantly.

3. Pour the soy milk into a blender and blend while adding the agar mixture. If you are using all of the oil substitute to be used immediately in a salad dressing, add all the other dressing ingredients, blend until smooth, and chill for 45 minutes. If making it to have on hand, store it in a closed container in the refrigerator without adding the other dressing ingredients, and use it in place of oil in salad dressings.

TOFU SOUR CREAM

Makes 1 cup

Use as a condiment in place of sour cream.

1 C regular Japanese (soft) tofu, well drained

1 T fresh lemon juice

1 tsp. vinegar

⅛ tsp. salt

⅛ tsp. honey

½ tsp. nutritional yeast

Place all the ingredients in a blender or food processor and blend until well blended. Chill.

AVOCADO SOUR CREAM

Makes 1 cup

Use this as a condiment in place of real sour cream. Place a dab of it in chilled borscht or on refried beans.

1 *large ripe (green, not darkened) avocado, peeled and pitted*

2 *tsp. fresh lemon juice*
1 *tsp. vinegar*
⅛ *tsp. salt*

Mash the avocado well with a fork, breaking up all the lumps. Add the rest of the ingredients and beat with a fork until well blended. Chill.

BARBECUE SAUCE

Makes about 1¼ cups

1 *tsp. cold-pressed olive oil*
½ *onion, chopped*
½ *C tomato paste*
½ *C apple juice*
1 *tsp. dry mustard*
⅛ *tsp. cinnamon*

¼ *tsp. black pepper, ground*
½ *clove garlic, chopped*
¼ *tsp. paprica*
2 *T natural soy sauce*
¼ *C vinegar*
1 *T honey*

1. Heat the oil in a saucepan. Add the onions and cook, covered, until they are golden.

2. Combine the tomato paste and apple juice and blend well. Add this and all remaining ingredients, except the honey, to the onions. Simmer for 20 minutes. If it gets too thick add a little water. The sauce should be thick at the end of the cooking time.

3. Remove from heat and stir in the honey.

4. Blend until smooth in a blender or food processor.

EDEN CHEESY SAUCE

Makes 2 cups

The chefs at Eden Foods created this creamy cheese-like topping using Edensoy Original flavor. Use it as a topping for pizza or as a cheese sauce over macaroni or steamed vegetables.

1½ C soy milk
2 blocks (⅓ package) plain mochi, cut into ¼-inch pieces

1 tsp. salt
½ tsp. dried oregano
1 clove garlic, pressed

Combine all the ingredients in a small saucepan. Bring to a boil and simmer until mochi is completely melted, 5 to 10 minutes. Stir frequently to prevent scorching. Dribble the warm sauce over the top of a pizza 10 minutes before the pizza is completely baked or toss it with warm, cooked macaroni or vegetables.

DILL SAUCE

1 C Mayo Spread I or II (pages 87, 88)

1 tsp. dried dill

Mix the Mayo Spread and dried dill together with a spoon and refrigerate at least 3 hours before using.

This sauce is particularly delicious as a dressing for potato salad.

SAUCE VERTE

Makes 1 cup

This dressing is ideal for a cold vegetable salad.

2 T chopped parsley

2 T chopped chives

2 T chopped watercress or chopped mustard greens

1 C Mayo Spread I or II (pages 87, 88) or mayonnaise

Chop all the greens together until they are very finely minced. Stir them into the Mayo Spread and chill for 1 hour.

MUSHROOM HORSERADISH SAUCE

Makes 1½ cups

1 tsp. natural olive oil

½ onion, finely chopped

¼ tsp. salt

1 clove garlic, finely chopped

6 medium mushrooms, sliced

1 C water

2 T red wine

2 tsp. prepared horseradish

1 T natural soy sauce

pepper to taste

¼ tsp. paprika

1. Heat the oil in a saucepan and add the onion. Sprinkle salt over the onion, cover, and cook over medium heat until the onion is golden. The salt will release water from the onion and it will stew in its own juice.

2. Add the garlic and mushrooms and cook, covered, for 3 minutes. Add all the other ingredients and cook, covered, for 20 minutes more. Serve over Pecan Herb Loaf (page 150), mashed potatoes, or vegetables such as green beans, zucchini, or summer squash.

PEANUT SAUCE

Makes 2 cups

This delicious sauce from the Basil Street Cafe restaurant in Leucadia, California, turns simple vegetables into an Oriental feast.

2 small onions, chopped
2 cloves garlic, minced
1 tsp. peanut oil
½ C peanut butter
2 T miso
1 T toasted sesame oil
4 T soy sauce
2 T ground cumin
2 T honey

2 T ground ginger
2 tsp. paprika
¼ tsp. ground cayenne
   pepper
1½ C Vegetable Stock (page
   110) or vegetarian stock
   base prepared
   according to package
   directions

1. Sauté the onions and garlic in the peanut oil until the onions are tender.

2. Transfer to a blender or food processor. Add the remaining sauce ingredients and blend until creamy.

3. Return to the sauté pan and bring to a simmer. Serve immediately over tempeh, steamed or stir-fried vegetables, or noodles.

WILD MUSHROOM GRAVY

Makes 1½ cups

This gravy can be made with any kind of dried wild mushroom such as shitaki, porcini, or oyster. They each have a slightly different taste, so try them all and choose your favorite.

4 *dried wild mushrooms (2 inches in diameter; use more or fewer mushrooms depending on size)*

1 *C boiling water*

1 *tsp. cold-pressed olive oil*

½ *onion, finely chopped*

1 *garlic clove, finely chopped*

½ *tsp. oregano*

2 *T natural soy sauce*

2 *T white wine*

1 *T cold-pressed olive oil*

2 *T whole wheat pastry flour*

salt and pepper to taste

1. Break up each mushroom into three or four pieces, including the stems. Place in a small bowl and pour boiling water over them. Let stand for 30 minutes.

2. Heat 1 teaspoon of the olive oil in a small skillet, add the onion, and cook until golden. Add the garlic and oregano and cook for 1 minute more. Add the mushrooms and soaking water, soy sauce, and wine. Cover and simmer for 40 minutes. Add salt and pepper to taste.

3. Pour off the liquid into a measuring cup and add water to this stock to make 1 cup. Return it to the skillet.

4. Remove the mushrooms and let them cool until they can be handled. Cut away the stems and discard, then slice the mushrooms and put aside.

5. Pass the stock through a sieve to purée and set aside.

6. In a saucepan, heat the remaining olive oil, add the flour, and stir continuously for 1 minute. Remove from the heat and add the stock all at once, whisking briskly. If any lumps appear, beat with an egg-beater until they are dissolved. Bring to a boil, whisking, and cook for 2 minutes. Add the sliced mushrooms. Serve over plain pasta, mashed potatoes, tofu, or tempeh.

10

ENTRÉES FOR
THE MEAT LOVER

MARINATED TEMPEH

Serves four (four slices)

Tempeh is lower in fat and higher in fiber than its relative, tofu, and has a distinctive taste that varies according to brand and ingredients added to it. Most tempeh is made from soy beans only, but tempeh made from a mixture of beans and grains is also available and often has a milder flavor.

½ lb. tempeh (one package)   *Tempeh Marinade (page 143)*

1. Cut the tempeh in half widthwise. With a sharp knife cut each slice into two thinner slices so that they are the same length and width and half the thickness.

2. Place the tempeh slices in a sealed container with the marinade for two to four days, unless the rec-ipe you are using states otherwise. Make sure that all the slices are covered by the marinade by turning the container over every day.

3. Remove the tempeh from the marinade, drain, and proceed according to the recipe.

MARINATED TOFU

Makes 8 to 10 slices

1 *lb. firm Chinese tofu*   *Tempeh Marinade (page 143)*

1. Drain the tofu and cut into ¼-inch-thick to ⅓-inch-thick slices. Place the slices side by side on a clean, absorbent kitchen towel. Cover with another towel. Place a large book on top and allow the tofu to drain for 30 minutes.

2. Place the tofu slices and marinade in a sealed container and marinate for two to four days, unless the recipe you are using states otherwise. Make sure that all the slices are covered by the marinade by turning the container over every day.

3. Remove the tofu from the marinade, drain, and proceed according to the recipe.

BARBECUED TOFU OR TEMPEH

Serves four to six people

1 *lb. Marinated Tofu (page 142) or 1 lb. Marinated Tempeh (page 141)*

Cold-pressed olive oil (optional)

Barbecue sauce (page 135)

1. Preheat the broiler.

2. Drain the marinated tofu. Brush the tofu very lightly with oil and barbecue sauce and grill under the broiler until browned on one side. Turn over and grill the other side.

3. Serve with Malibu Chile (page 22) or Apple-Honey Baked Beans (page 223), or serve on a whole wheat hamburger bun with sliced tomatoes, lettuce, and all your favorite condiments.

TEMPEH MARINADE

Makes enough to marinate 1 lb. of tempeh or tofu.

1 tsp. cold-pressed olive oil

1 small onion, finely chopped

3 garlic cloves, finely chopped

6 mushrooms, one week old, thinly sliced, or 3 dried shitake mushrooms, broken, stems included, and soaked for 30 minutes in ¼ C water

¾ C water

¼ C apple juice

1 tsp. oregano

¼ tsp. basil

¼ tsp. tarragon

1 T vinegar

½ C red wine

⅓ C natural soy sauce

dash of nutmeg

⅛ tsp. pepper

½ tsp. salt

Heat the oil in a saucepan. Add the onion and cook until golden. Add the garlic and cook for 1 minute more. Add all the other ingredients and simmer, covered, for 30 minutes. Include the soaking water if shitake mushrooms are used. Strain the marinade through a very fine sieve or a double thickness of cheesecloth.

TERIYAKI TOFU

Serves four

In taste and texture, this dish is reminiscent of chicken.

1 *lb. Chinese tofu, firm*

¼ *C Braggs Aminos (Soy sauce may be used for a slightly different taste.)*

2 *T nutritional yeast*

2 *tsp. garlic powder*

2 *tsp. onion powder*

8 *bamboo skewers*

¼ *C teriyaki sauce*

2 *T cold-pressed olive oil*

1. Preheat the oven to 350°F. Cut the tofu into strips about ¼ inch thick and ¾ inch wide. Press the slices gently in a clean kitchen towel to expel excess water. Arrange on a lightly oiled baking dish so that the pieces do not touch.

2. Brush liberally with Braggs Aminos. Sprinkle liberally with nutritional yeast, garlic powder, and onion powder.

3. Bake for 40 minutes but do not allow it to scorch. Let cool for 5 minutes.

4. Thread lengthwise onto the bamboo skewers. Return to the baking dish. Brush with teriyaki sauce and a little olive oil. Heat under the broiler for 5 minutes. Do not allow to burn.

5. Serve on a bed of brown rice as a main dish, or with Chinese mustard as an hors d'oeuvre.

POLYNESIAN TOFU

Serves six

If you like Hawaiian chicken, you'll love this dish.

SAUCE

3 *tsp. arrowroot powder or kuzu*

1 *C unsweetened pineapple juice or apple juice*

1 *T honey*

2 *T white vinegar*

2 *T soy sauce*

salt to taste

2 *tsp. cold-pressed olive oil*

½ *onion, cut into bite-size pieces*

1 *clove garlic, finely chopped*

2 *stalks celery, sliced diagonally into ½-inch pieces*

1 *green pepper, seeds and membranes removed, cut into bite-size pieces*

1 *T very thinly sliced fresh ginger*

2 *T slivered almonds*

2 *C ripe fresh pineapple chunks, or 2 C unsweetened canned pineapple chunks, drained (reserve juice for use in the sauce)*

1 *lb. firm Chinese tofu prepared as Teriyaki Tofu steps 1 through 3 (page 144)*

1. To prepare the sauce, dissolve the arrowroot in 2 tablespoons pineapple juice or apple juice. Add the honey and a little more juice, if necessary, and stir until the honey is dissolved. Mix in the remaining juice and all other sauce ingredients and set aside.

2. Heat the oil in a large skillet or wok. Add the onion and garlic and sauté for 2 minutes over medium heat. Add the celery, pepper, and ginger and sauté for 3 minutes. Add the almonds and pineapple and cook for 4 minutes or until the vegetables are tender but still crisp.

3. Add the sauce to the vegetables and cook, stirring, for 2 minutes or until the sauce thickens and becomes clear.

4. Adjust the seasoning.

5. Just before serving mix in the tofu. Serve on a bed of brown rice.

TOFU PIQUANT

Serves four

COOKED TOFU

1 lb. firm Chinese tofu

4 T Braggs Aminos or
    natural soy sauce

1 tsp. garlic powder

1 tsp. onion powder

PIQUANT

1 tsp. cold-pressed olive oil

2 T chopped shallots

2 T capers

½ T (5 sprigs) finely
    chopped parsley

3 T fresh lemon juice

2 T natural soy sauce

1 T water

¼ C lightly steamed green
    peas (frozen, if fresh
    are not available)

1. To cook the tofu, preheat the oven to 350°F.

2. Cut the tofu into slices ¼ to ⅓ inch thick. Press gently between clean kitchen towels to expel excess water.

3. Lay the slices in a single layer in an oiled baking dish. Cover each slice with 2 teaspoons of the Braggs Aminos or soy sauce and sprinkle liberally with the garlic and onion powders.

4. Bake for 40 minutes. (If the slices start to blacken, remove from the oven, lower the heat, wait 5 minutes, and return to the oven.)

5. To make the piquant, place the olive oil in a medium skillet and heat. Add the shallots and sauté for 3 minutes. Add the capers, parsley, lemon juice, 2 tablespoons of soy sauce, water, and peas and cook, covered, for 5 minutes. Add the cooked tofu and cook for 1 minute more.

6. Serve on a bed of steamed brown rice. Garnish with parsley sprigs and lemon slices.

TOFU RIBS

Serves four

These are a tasty treat as an appetizer or as part of the main course. They go especially well as part of a Chinese meal.

1 *lb. Marinated Tofu (page 142)*

2 *T cold-pressed vegetable oil*

8 *bamboo skewers*

Barbecue Sauce (page 135)

1. Preheat the oven to 300°F.

2. Cut the marinated tofu slices lengthwise into three strips per slice.

3. Brush the tofu slices on all sides with oil and lay them, side by side, in a dish. The slices should not touch. Bake for 40 minutes.

4. Remove from the oven and let cool for 5 minutes. Pass bamboo skewers carefully through the width of each slice. Five to six slices will fit onto one skewer without touching. Cover with barbecue sauce and preheat the broiler.

5. Broil 6 inches from the heat for about 5 minutes, turn over, and repeat. The tofu can become dark, but scorching will make it bitter.

GRILLED TOFU WITH SUMMER VEGETABLES

Serves four to six

In Los Angeles there is a small chain of natural food markets called Mrs. Gooch's. Every day, in their deli section, they put out freshly made salads, entrees, and desserts. This dish is a favorite of ours.

1 *16-oz. package firm Chinese tofu, cubed*

¾ *C natural teriyaki sauce*

1 *red bell pepper, cut into 1-inch pieces*

1 *green bell pepper, cut into 1-inch pieces*

1 *large white onion, cut into 1-inch pieces*

12 *large mushrooms, halved*

12 *bamboo skewers, soaked in water for 1 hour*

2 *T cold-pressed canola oil or safflower oil*

2 *C Barbecue Sauce (page 135)*

1. Combine the tofu and teriyaki sauce in a sealed plastic bag. Freeze overnight and thaw the next day. Turn the bag once or twice during the thawing process. Reserve the marinade.

2. Place the tofu, peppers, onion, and mushrooms on skewers, alternating the order, beginning and ending with tofu. Combine the oil with the reserved marinade and brush on the tofu and vegetables. Place on a grill and brown on all sides. Brush on barbecue sauce and grill a while longer. Serve with Rosemary Brown Rice Pilaf (page 195).

JAPANESE EGGPLANT AND TOFU ROMANO

Serves six

This delicious dish is elegant and satisfying, an ideal entrée to serve to nonvegetarian friends. And, like many Italian dishes, it not only keeps well in the refrigerator for several days but is actually better the next day, so make plenty for leftovers.

TOFU

1 *lb. marinated tofu, drained*

2 *T cold-pressed olive oil*

EGGPLANT

6 *medium-to-large Japanese eggplants*

2 *T soy sauce*

2 *T lemon juice*

2 *T water*

2 *T cold-pressed olive oil*

4 *C Sesame Tomato Sauce (page 162)*

1. Preheat the oven to 350°F.

2. Brush the marinated tofu slices lightly with 2 tablespoons of the olive oil and bake for 30 minutes.

3. Wash the eggplants and cut off the tops. Do not peel. Cut lengthwise into ¼-inch slices. Discard the pieces that are mostly peel.

4. Mix the soy sauce, lemon juice, water, and the remaining olive oil. On a lightly oiled baking sheet lay out the eggplant in a single layer. Brush the tops generously with the soy sauce mixture. Turn each piece over and brush the other side. Bake for 10 minutes or until the eggplant becomes limp. Don't overcook or it will be mushy. If the eggplant becomes dry, brush again with the soy sauce mixture.

5. Spread a thin layer of Sesame Tomato Sauce on the bottom of a baking dish and arrange the baked tofu in a single layer on top of it. Completely cover with sauce, then lay eggplant strips side by side over the sauce using all the eggplant. Cover with the remainder of the sauce.

6. Bake, uncovered, for 30 minutes. Cool for 10 minutes before serving.

PECAN HERB LOAF

Serves six

This great alternative to meat loaf has the taste and the texture to satisfy the fussiest meat loaf maven. Make enough for leftovers because it's delicious served cold on sandwiches or crumbled in pita bread.

LOAF

½ onion, finely chopped

1 tsp. cold-pressed olive oil

8 medium mushrooms, finely chopped

6 large garlic cloves, finely chopped

½ C chopped pecans

½ C chopped almonds

¼ C chia seeds (if unavailable use ½ C hulled sesame seeds)

2 T raw soy flour

2 T arrowroot powder

4 T nutritional yeast

1½ tsp. salt

¼ tsp. ground black pepper

½ tsp. basil

¼ tsp. oregano

¼ tsp. savory

¾ tsp. garlic powder

20 oz. firm Chinese tofu

5 T raw tahini

SAUCE

½ onion, finely chopped

1 T cold-pressed olive oil

2 14-oz. cans chopped tomatoes

½ T soy sauce

¼ tsp. ground black pepper

¼ tsp. garlic powder

½ tsp. basil

1. Sauté the onion in olive oil over medium heat for 3 minutes. Add the mushrooms and cook, covered for 5 minutes. Add the garlic and cook for 2 minutes more.

2. Place the pecans and almonds in a food processor or blender. Using short strokes at medium speed, chop the nuts until they have the texture of very coarse corn meal.

3. Combine the nuts, chia seeds, soy flour, arrowroot, yeast, salt, pepper, basil, oregano, savory, and garlic powder in a large mixing bowl

and mix well.

4. Place the tofu, half at a time, in a clean dish cloth. Collect the corners and wring tightly to expel as much water as possible. Do not use cheesecloth since the holes would allow the tofu to pass through. The tofu will crumble. Break up any large pieces that remain.

5. Combine the tofu thoroughly with the onion-mushroom mixture and tahini. Add to the dry ingredients and combine well (using your hands works especially well).

6. Press firmly into an oiled loaf pan (preferably glass) and bake at 350°F for 1 hour.

7. While the loaf is baking, prepare the sauce. Sauté the onion in olive oil over medium heat for 7 minutes. Add all the other ingredients and cook, covered, for 30 minutes and uncovered for 15 minutes more.

8. Remove the loaf from the heat and let stand, covered, for 15 minutes. Turn out onto a serving dish, cover with sauce, and garnish with sprigs of parsley. To serve, slice and cover each slice with sauce.

NOTE. For special occasions substitute Mushroom Horseradish Sauce (page 137) for the sauce shown above and serve with mashed potatoes.

PECAN HERB BURGERS

Makes 10 to 12 patties

1 *recipe Pecan Herb Loaf (page 150), omitting the sauce*

1. Follow instructions 1 through 5.

2. Press the mixture firmly into patties.

3. Bake at 350°F in an oiled baking dish for 35 minutes or until the patties are firm and browned. Serve on warm, whole wheat burger buns with lettuce, tomatoes, and your favorite condiments. Baked patties can be eaten immediately, frozen for future use, or spread with barbecue sauce and barbecued for 10 minutes.

Boulettes
(Spaghetti Balls)

Makes about 20

In France meatballs are called *boulettes* and they contain all sorts of ingredients, not just meat. Here's our version.

1 *recipe Pecan Herb Loaf*
(page 150), omitting the
sauce

Tomato Sauce (page 163)

1. Follow instructions 1 through 5 for Pecan Herb Loaf.

2. Roll the mixture into balls.

3. Bake at 350°F in an oiled baking dish for 35 minutes or until the boulettes are firm and browned. Serve on pasta and cover with Tomato Sauce.

VARIATIONS. For a Mediterranean flavor, place a pitted Greek olive in the center of each ball and bake as directed. For a South Seas flavor, place a small chunk of ripe pineapple in the center of each ball, bake, and serve with sweet and sour sauce. Try your own ideas.

EASY TOFU BURGERS

Makes 4 large patties

1 *lb. firm Chinese tofu*
¼ *C raw soy flour*
2 *T whole wheat flour*
2 *T arrowroot powder*
2 *tsp. paprika*
½ *tsp. garlic powder*
¼ *tsp. black pepper*

¼ *tsp. ginger powder*
3 *T natural soy sauce*
¼ *small onion, very finely chopped*
1 *green onion, very finely chopped*
2 *T cold-pressed vegetable oil for cooking*

1. Drain the tofu. Wrap in a clean nonterry kitchen towel and wring out excess water. The tofu will crumble.

2. Combine the soy flour, whole wheat flour, arrowroot powder, paprika, garlic powder, pepper, and ginger powder and mix well.

3. Mix the tofu, soy sauce, onion, and green onion. Add the dry ingredients and mix well. Knead with your hands until all the ingredients are thoroughly blended and the mixture holds together. Let stand for 20 minutes. Form into patties.

4. Heat the oil in a skillet. Add the patties and, over medium heat, cook for 7 minutes. Turn over and cook for 7 minutes more. Serve on whole wheat hamburger buns with lettuce and tomatoes, or serve like Salisbury steak. Also, try making these into balls to serve with spaghetti.

EASY, EASY BURGERS

Makes 5 burgers

We always try to have tempeh or tofu marinating in the refrigerator so we can put together burgers in a hurry.

Marinated Tempeh (page 141) or Marinated Tofu (page 142)

1 *T cold-pressed olive oil*

5 *whole wheat hamburger buns*

5 *slices large, ripe tomato (2 slices per person if tomatoes are small)*

lettuce

sliced pickles

Mayo Spread I or II (pages 87, 88)

catsup

mustard

1. Blot the slices of tofu or tempeh gently with a clean paper towel. Oil the bottom of a skillet, heat, and add the tempeh or tofu in a single layer. Cook over medium heat until the undersides are browned. Loosen the tofu or tempeh often with a spatula while it cooks since it will have the tendency to stick. Turn the slices over and brown the second side.

2. Serve on hamburger buns with tomato slices, lettuce, sliced pickles, Mayo Spread, catsup, mustard, or your favorite condiments.

NEW AGE ITALIAN SAUSAGE I

Makes 10 sausages

Serve these sausages with spaghetti, in sandwiches, or on pizza. They will liven up any dish. For a Mexican flavor omit the basil, oregano, and savory and use cumin and chili powder instead. A dash of cayenne pepper will make the sausage spicy hot. Prepare this dish a day before you need it.

¼ lb. Marinated Tempeh (page 141), marinated for no more than 24 hours

½ lb. Marinated Tofu (page 142), marinated for no more than 24 hours

1 T chopped fresh parsley

1 T chopped fresh basil or 1 tsp. dry basil

¼ tsp. oregano

¼ tsp. honey

2 tsp. paprika

½ tsp. ground black pepper

1 tsp. garlic powder

¼ tsp. savory

1. Blot the marinated tempeh and marinated tofu slices several times with paper towels to remove all excess marinade. Crumble them up and put them in a food processor (if you are using a blender, chop the tempeh and tofu until very fine before blending).

2. Add all the other ingredients and chop until fine, about 45 seconds. The mixture should be well blended and easily formed into sausages. If you're using a blender you'll need to blend for a longer time.

3. Preheat the oven to 350°F. Form into thumb-size sausages, pressing to make them as compact as possible. Bake for 40 minutes. Do not allow the sausages to blacken.

New Age Italian Sausage II

Makes approximately 10 sausages

1 *lb. Marinated Tofu (page 142)*

4 *T whole wheat flour*

4 *T gluten flour or 4 T whole wheat flour*

2 *T dry whole wheat bread crumbs*

1 *T chopped parsley*

¼ *tsp. pepper*

½ *tsp. basil*

½ *tsp. oregano*

½ *tsp. savory*

2 *tsp. paprika*

1 *garlic clove, pressed*

½ *C chopped almonds*

1 *T cold-pressed olive oil*

1. Remove the tofu from the marinade and crumble. Reserve the liquid in case the sausages are too dry. Mix the marinated tofu with the flours, bread crumbs, parsley, pepper, basil, oregano, savory, paprika, and garlic. Place in a food processor or blender and chop for 30 seconds. Add the almonds and chop for 30 seconds more.

2. Take a little of the dough and press it into a sausage. If it forms easily and does not crumble, go ahead and form the rest into sausages about 2 inches long and ¾ inch in diameter. If the sausage crumbles, add a little marinade.

3. Heat oil in a large skillet and sauté the sausages until golden brown on all sides.

ITALIAN SAUSAGES AND PEPPERS

Serves eight

Like most Italian dishes, this one is better the day after it is made, so make plenty for leftovers. It also tastes great on a hero sandwich.

1 *tsp. cold-pressed olive oil*

2 *medium onions, halved and sliced*

4 *cloves garlic, thinly sliced*

⅛ to ¼ *tsp. ground black pepper*

½ *tsp. basil*

½ *tsp. oregano*

dash of cayenne

3 *green peppers, membranes and seeds removed, cut into strips*

3 *red peppers, membranes and seeds removed, cut into strips*

1 *can (about 14 oz.) Italian tomatoes, chopped*

salt to taste

8 *New Age Italian Sausages I or II (pages 155, 156) cut into ½-inch chunks*

1. Heat the oil in a large skillet. Add the onions and cook slowly until limp. Add the garlic, pepper, basil, oregano, and cayenne and cook for 2 minutes more. Add the peppers, tomatoes, and salt and cook, covered, over low heat for 60 minutes. Fast cooking over high heat will make the peppers bitter.

2. Add salt to taste and cook, uncovered, for 10 minutes. The sauce should be thick but not watery or dry.

3. Stir in the sausages and cook for 2 minutes more. Add more salt and pepper if desired.

4. Serve immediately on a bed of whole wheat pasta.

SPICY TEMPEH STIR-FRY

Serves four

This exotic treat was created at the Basil Street Cafe restaurant in Leucadia, near San Diego, California. It is the ideal centerpiece for a meal with an Oriental flavor.

COOKED TEMPEH

¼ *C cold-pressed peanut oil*

¼ *C soy sauce*

8 *oz. soy tempeh cut into bite-size cubes*

STIR-FRY

½ *T cold-pressed peanut oil*

½ *T toasted sesame oil*

½ *small onion, sliced*

4 *C assorted sliced vegetables (carrots, bok choy, red cabbage, broccoli)*

¼ *C Easy Vegetable Stock (page 110) or vegetarian broth base prepared according to package directions*

4 *T soy sauce*

1 *T miso*

cooked tempeh

2 *C Peanut Sauce (page 138)*

1. To prepare the tempeh, whisk ¼ cup of the peanut oil and soy sauce together and toss with the tempeh.

2. Bake 10 minutes at 425°F. Turn the cubes and bake an additional 10 minutes or until browned.

3. To prepare the stir-fry, heat the oils in a wok. Add the onion and stir-fry for 2 minutes over high heat. Add the other vegetables and cook for 1 minute more, stirring constantly.

4. Add the stock, soy sauce, miso, and cooked tempeh. Lower the heat, cover, and cook for 3 to 5 minutes. The vegetables should be tender but crisp.

5. Top with Peanut Sauce and serve with steamed brown rice.

TOFU CACCIATORE

Serves four

1 lb. firm Chinese tofu

2 C water

1 tsp. cold-pressed olive oil

3 garlic cloves, minced

3 T tomato paste

¾ C Mushroom Stock (page 109) or any vegetarian stock

1 C canned tomatoes, chopped or 2 ripe tomatoes, chopped

⅓ lb. mushrooms, sliced

½ C dry white wine

1 T fresh chopped parsley

½ tsp. salt

½ bay leaf

¼ tsp. rosemary

¼ tsp. basil

⅛ tsp. white pepper

¼ tsp. black pepper

1. Drain the tofu and cut into ½-inch squares. Boil the water, add the tofu, and simmer for 5 minutes. Drain and discard the water.

2. In a large skillet heat the olive oil, add the garlic, and cook for 2 minutes.

3. In a small bowl, mix the tomato paste and mushroom stock and whisk until blended. Add this tomato mixture and all the other ingredients to the skillet. Bring to a boil, reduce the heat, and simmer, covered, for 20 minutes, stirring often. Uncover and simmer for 20 minutes more. Add a little water if the mixture gets too dry. Serve over whole wheat pasta.

11

PASTA, PIZZA, AND OTHER GRAIN ENTRÉES

PASTA PRIMAVERA

Serves four to six

When the colorful springtime vegetables ripen, it's time for Pasta Primavera, literally, springtime pasta. The colors are bright and cheerful and the taste is subtle and sweet. It's important that the vegetables be crisp.

1 *garlic clove, thinly sliced*

1 *T cold-pressed olive oil (use less to reduce fat)*

1 *lb. whole wheat shells*

10 *green beans*

¼ *C Easy Vegetable Stock (page 110) or any vegetarian broth*

2 *carrots, cut into matchsticks*

1 *yellow crookneck squash, halved lengthwise and sliced*

1 *C cauliflower florets, bite-size*

1 *C broccoli florets, bite-size*

½ *sweet red pepper, diced*

½ *C fresh peas*

¼ *tsp. salt*

⅛ *tsp. pepper*

1. Soak the garlic in the olive oil for 30 minutes. Discard the garlic and reserve the oil. Cook the shells according to the package directions.

2. Steam the green beans for 5 minutes. They will be just tender and still crisp. In a large skillet, heat the stock. Immediately add the car-

continued on next page

rots, squash, cauliflower, broccoli, red pepper, peas, salt, and pepper. Cover and cook for 5 minutes or until the vegetables are just tender.

3. Remove the shells from their cooking water with a slotted spoon.

Let them drain momentarily but don't allow them to become dry. Place in a large warm bowl, add the cooked vegetables and garlic oil, and toss. Serve immediately. To reheat, first add a tablespoon or two of water or broth.

SESAME TOMATO SAUCE

Makes 4 cups

This sauce is a pleasant alternative to traditional spaghetti sauces. It has a light and interesting taste.

1 *tsp. cold-pressed olive oil*

1 *medium onion, finely chopped*

2 *cloves garlic, chopped*

1 *28-oz. can of tomatoes, chopped*

½ *tsp. toasted sesame oil*

3 *T soy sauce*

3 *T barley malt syrup*

1 *tsp. dried basil*

dash of ginger

1. Heat the olive oil in a large skillet. Add the onion and garlic and cook, covered, over medium heat until the onion is limp and translucent, about 10 minutes. If the onion starts to brown, reduce the heat.

2. Add all the other ingredients and cook, covered, for 30 minutes. Remove the cover and cook for 10 minutes more to boil away excess liquid. The sauce will be chunky. If you prefer a smooth sauce, purée in a blender or pass through a strainer.

TOMATO SAUCE

Makes 5 cups

This easy sauce comes from Los Angeles chef Daniel LaBella. It's easy to make and has a bright taste. For dishes with their own distinctive taste such as Lasagna with Zucchini and Mushrooms (page 168), make the sauce as directed but omit the basil, oregano, and marjoram.

2 *tsp. cold-pressed olive oil*

½ *onion, finely chopped*

½ *tsp. dried basil*

½ *tsp. dried oregano*

¼ *tsp. marjoram*

2 *large garlic cloves,*
chopped

6 *oz. tomato paste*

28 *oz. canned* or *fresh*
tomatoes, chopped

1 *C water*

Salt and pepper

1. Place the oil in a large saucepan. Add the onion, basil, oregano, and marjoram and cook, covered, over medium heat until the onion is golden. Add the garlic and cook for 1 minute more. Remove the onion and garlic and reserve.

2. Place the tomato paste in the same saucepan and cook over medium heat for 5 minutes, stirring constantly.

3. Add the canned tomatoes and mash with a fork or potato masher.

If you prefer a creamier sauce, blend the tomatoes in a blender until smooth. Add the water and bring to a fast boil.

4. Reduce the heat. Add the reserved onion, garlic, salt, and pepper. Simmer, covered, for 1 hour, stirring occasionally.

NOTE. For thick sauce (if sauce is to be used for pizza), cook, uncovered, during the last half hour, stirring often to prevent burning.

Tomato Garbanzo Bean Sauce

Makes 4 cups

Left chunky, this sauce is used for Risotto with Tomatoes and Garbanzo Beans (page 185) and is ideal over lightly steamed vegetables and plain pasta. When it is blended until smooth, it makes a perfect sauce for pizzas and casseroles, with a sweet, almost ricotta taste.

2 *tsp. cold-pressed olive oil*

1 *small onion, finely chopped*

5 *parsley springs*

2 *garlic cloves*

4 *C cooked, or canned, or fresh tomatoes, chopped*

salt to taste

pepper to taste

1 *C cooked garbanzo beans, drained*

1. Heat the oil in a large skillet. Add the onion and cook slowly until translucent. Onions that are cooked slowly and are not allowed to burn become very sweet.

2. Chop the parsley and garlic together and add to the onion. Cook for 3 minutes. Add the tomatoes with their liquid, salt, and pepper. Bring to a boil and cook for 30 minutes. Add the garbanzo beans and cook for 10 minutes more.

3. If the sauce is to be smooth, blend in a food processor or a blender until smooth.

Pasta Dough

Makes about ⅔ lb. dry or 4 C cooked

Pasta is one of those things, like yeasted bread, that sounds complicated. Well, this dough is so easy to make, almost fool-proof, and so delicious that you may never buy pasta again.

1 C whole wheat pastry
  flour, passed through a
  fine tea strainer to
  remove coarse bran

¼ tsp. salt

¼ to ⅓ C water

1. Place the flour and salt in a mixing bowl. Slowly add the water, mixing until the dough becomes stiff enough to knead. Use only as much water as necessary to make an elastic dough. Knead the dough for 10 minutes, form into a ball, cover, and let stand at room temperature for 1 hour.

2. Roll out and follow directions for your favorite pasta found on the next few pages. If you have a pasta machine, follow the operating instructions.

FLAT NOODLES

Pasta Dough (page 164)

1. Cut the dough ball into two sections. On a floured board, roll out dough, adding enough flour so that the dough doesn't stick to the rolling pin or to the board. Roll until very thin and allow to dry for 1 hour.

2. Dust the dough lightly with flour and roll up. With a sharp knife, cut the roll into slices as wide as you want your noodles to be. The slices will unroll easily to form noodles. Lay one layer of noodles on a clean kitchen towel. Cover with another towel and repeat.

3. Cook the noodles in 5 quarts of rapidly boiling water to which ½ teaspoon salt and 1 tablespoon olive oil have been added. Cook about 5 minutes or until the noodles are *al dente*, just a little resistant to the bite.

CANNELONI OR MANICOTTI SHELLS

Serves four

Let your imagination run wild when you are deciding on the fillings. We have given a suggestion for manicotti (page 175) but that's just a start—don't forget that some of the best fillings were left over from last night's dinner.

Pasta Dough (page 164)

1. Cut the dough ball into two parts. On a floured board, roll out the dough into a thin rectangle, dusting with just enough flour to keep dough from sticking to the rolling pin or the board. Cut into rectangles about 4 by 4 inches for canneloni and 4 by 6 inches for manicotti.

2. Drop into a large amount of rapidly boiling water containing ⅓ teaspoon salt and 1 tablespoon olive oil. It is important that the water continue to boil rapidly. Cook the rectangles for about 5 minutes until *al dente,* then cool with cold water.

3. Remove the dough rectangles carefully from the water with an open spatula and place on a wet-towel-covered counter to drain.

4. Fill by spreading 1½ tablespoons of filling along one edge of the pasta (the longer edge, if making canneloni), then roll up starting at that edge. Bake, seam side up, following the directions on page 175.

Spinach Pecan Ravioli

Makes 12 ravioli

Pasta Dough (page 164)

1 tsp. cold-pressed olive oil

¼ onion, minced

1 large garlic clove, crushed

1 bunch spinach, washed twice and coarsely chopped

½ tsp. salt

¼ tsp. pepper

¼ C chopped pecans

2 C Tomato Sauce (page 163)

1. Prepare the Pasta Dough through step 1 as directed.

2. Heat the oil in a large skillet. Add the onion and cook, covered, until golden. Turn off the heat. Add the garlic and mix well. Add the spinach, salt, and pepper, cover, and cook until the spinach is wilted. Remove the cover, add the chopped pecans, and cook until all the liquid has evaporated.

3. Cut the dough into two sections. On a floured board, roll the dough into a thin rectangle. Set aside. Do the same with the second part of the dough.

4. Place small mounds of filling, about 1 teaspoon, 1½ inches apart on one dough rectangle. Cover with the second dough rectangle. Press down with the side of your little finger between the mounds. With a knife or pastry cutter, cut into individual ravioli. If a knife was used, seal the edges by pressing lightly with the tines of a fork.

5. Line up the ravioli on a floured towel.

6. In a large pot, boil 7 quarts of water containing ½ teaspoon salt and 1 tablespoon olive oil. The water should continue boiling rapidly. Place the ravioli in the water one at a time and cook for 10 minutes. Gently remove from the water with a slotted spoon and place in a colander to drain. Transfer to a large warm bowl and cover with tomato sauce, making sure that the sauce coats each ravioli.

Lasagna with Zucchini and Mushrooms

Serves four

This lasagna was inspired by the late Pierre Carretta, who for twenty-six years was the chef and chief source of good conversation at Pierre's Place in the old Brentwood Market in Los Angeles. His original version contained meat and cheese, so we have taken some liberties with the recipe. But the flair is all his. It can be made with packaged noodles. However, making the pasta yourself is not much more work than cooking up the ready-made noodles, and the difference is discernable.

1½ recipe Pasta Dough (page 164) or ½ lb. packaged lasagna noodles, cooked to package directions

LIGHT SAUCE

2⅔ T whole wheat pastry flour

1 C soy milk

¼ tsp. salt

dash of garlic

dash of nutmeg

1 tsp. fresh lemon juice

ZUCCHINI FILLING

2 tsp. cold-pressed olive oil

2 medium zucchini, sliced

2 cloves garlic, crushed

salt to taste

MUSHROOM FILLING

2 tsp. cold-pressed olive oil

½ lb. mushrooms, sliced

2 cloves garlic, crushed

1 T chopped fresh basil or ¼ tsp. dried basil

salt to taste

3 C Tomato Sauce (page 163), chunky, omit basil, oregano, and marjoram

1. Prepare the dough as indicated in the recipe. Set aside for 1 hour.

2. To prepare the light sauce, place the flour in a small saucepan

and gradually add the soy milk, whisking constantly. Add all the other light sauce ingredients and bring to a boil, stirring constantly. Cook for 2 minutes, continuing to stir. The sauce will be thick. Set aside.

3. To prepare the zucchini filling, heat the oil in a skillet. Add the zucchini, garlic, and salt and cook, covered, until the zucchini is tender but not mushy. If there is liquid left in the pan, remove the cover and cook for 1 minute to evaporate. Set aside.

4. To prepare the mushroom filling, heat the oil in a skillet, add the mushrooms, garlic, basil, and salt. Cook for 5 minutes or until the mushrooms are tender. Set aside.

5. Cut the pasta dough into four equal parts. On a floured board, roll each part into a rectangle about 10 by 6 inches.

6. Spread several tablespoons of Tomato Sauce in the bottom of a 9-by-5-inch loaf pan. (If you are doubling the recipe, use a 2½-inch-deep lasagna pan.) Place one sheet of noodle dough over the sauce or cover with one layer of cooked, packaged noodles. Divide the zucchini into two parts and spread one part evenly on the noodle. Cover with Tomato Sauce and another sheet of pasta. Spread all but ¼ cup of the light sauce and cover with mushrooms. Repeat with another layer of noodle, zucchini, and Tomato Sauce. Cover with the last sheet of pasta topped with Tomato Sauce. Shake the pan gently to settle the ingredients. Make sure the Tomato Sauce fills any holes in the corners and covers all the pasta. Dribble the remaining light sauce over the Tomato Sauce. Bake, covered, at 350°F for 35 minutes.

POTATO GNOCCHI

Serves four to six

Gnocchi are little dumplings that are eaten like pasta. Flour gnocchi are good, but potato gnocchi are superb.

2 *lb. large baking potatoes (about 3)*

1 *C whole wheat pastry flour*

½ *tsp. salt*

2 *C pasta sauce of your choice*

1. Steam the potatoes in their skins until tender. When they are cool enough to handle, peel and mash. Immediately add the flour and salt. Knead on a lightly floured board until smooth. Sprinkle on a little more flour if the dough sticks.

2. Form into rolls about the thickness of your thumb. Cut into ¾-inch sections and press down lightly with a fork.

3. Bring a large pot of lightly salted water to a boil. Add the gnocchi and boil until they rise to the top, about 5 minutes. Like all pasta, gnocchi should not be crowded in the pot, so cook them in several batches if necessary. Drain and place in a warm bowl.

4. Mix the gnocchi with enough sauce to completely coat them. Extra sauce can be added at the table according to taste.

Sweet Potato Gnocchi with Apple-Orange Tomato Sauce

Serves four to six

This odd combination of ingredients yields a deliciously bright taste that will end night-meal boredom. Serve it with a large mixed green salad in a simple vinaigrette dressing and steamed green beans, snap peas, or fresh peas.

THE GNOCCHI

2 lb. sweet potatoes (about 2 large)

1 C whole wheat pastry flour

½ tsp. salt

THE SAUCE

2 tsp. cold-pressed olive oil

1 onion, finely chopped

1 sweet apple, peeled, cored, and chopped

½ green pepper, diced

½ tsp. salt

3 C cooked, or canned, or fresh tomatoes, chopped

1 tsp. fresh grated orange peel

1. Prepare the sweet potato gnocchi according to instructions 1 and 2 for Potato Gnocchi (page 170). Since sweet potatoes can be stringy, mash by passing through a ricer, or, if mashing by hand, chop first. Cover and set aside until ready to boil.

2. To prepare the sauce, heat the oil in a large skillet. Add the onion and cook very slowly, without browning, until translucent. Slow cooking will make the onion sweet. Add the apple, green pepper, and salt and cook, covered, for 10 minutes. Add the tomatoes and orange peel and cook, covered, for 20 minutes. Uncover and cook for 5 minutes more.

3. Boil the sweet potato gnocchi according to directions for Potato Gnocchi.

4. Place the cooked sweet potato gnocchi in a warm bowl, add the sauce, and toss lightly.

NEAPOLITAN
PEPPERS AND PASTA

Serves four

Make plenty for leftovers because this is great reheated in sandwiches, in canneloni, or in pita bread.

2 *tsp. cold-pressed olive oil*

1 *onion, quartered and sliced*

3 *garlic cloves, crushed*

3 *sweet red peppers, seeds and membranes removed, cut into strips ¼ inch wide*

3 *green bell peppers, seeds and membranes removed, cut into strips ¼ inch wide*

1½ *T soy sauce*

¼ *tsp. ground black pepper*

pinch of cayenne

1 *C cooked or canned tomatoes, finely chopped (or use tomato sauce)*

1 *lb. whole wheat pasta, cooked according to package directions, or homemade pasta*

1. In a large skillet heat the oil. Add the onion and cook over medium heat until the onion is lightly browned.

2. Add the garlic, peppers, soy sauce, black pepper, and cayenne and cook, covered, for 7 minutes. Add the tomatoes or tomato sauce. Cook, covered, at low heat for 50 minutes. The peppers should be very tender but not mushy. If the peppers and sauce start sticking to the bottom of the pan, cover the skillet and turn off the heat for 3 minutes. This will allow you to stir the sauce off the bottom.

3. Serve over the pasta.

SPAGHETTI WITH TOMATOES AND BASIL

Serves four

1 *tsp. cold-pressed olive oil*

¼ *onion, finely chopped*

8 *cloves garlic, crushed*

1 *lb. fresh Rome tomatoes, chopped*

12 *fresh large basil leaves, chopped*

salt to taste

1 *lb. whole wheat spaghetti, cooked according to package directions, or homemade pasta*

Heat the oil in a large skillet. Add the onion and sauté until it is transparent. Add the garlic, tomatoes, basil leaves, and salt. Cook, covered, stirring occasionally, for 20 minutes. Serve over spaghetti.

LENTILS AND NOODLES

Serves eight

This dish is hearty, quick, and easy and it's especially satisfying in the wintertime. Put it in a wide-mouth thermos for a school lunch or serve it with a green salad, vegetables, and whole wheat bread for dinner.

1 *tsp. cold-pressed vegetable oil*

1 *large onion, chopped*

10 *C water*

2 *C lentils*

5 *large ripe tomatoes, chopped, with juices reserved*

1 *tsp. salt*

3 *T Braggs Aminos*

1 *lb. whole wheat elbow macaroni or shells*

1. Heat the oil in the bottom of a large pot. Add the onion and cook, covered, until the onion is tender. Add the water, lentils, and tomatoes and their juices. Bring to a boil and cook, covered, for 20 to 25 minutes. Stir often to prevent sticking.

2. Add the salt, Braggs Aminos, and macaroni and cook another 10 minutes or until noodles are tender. Stir often to prevent sticking.

MANICOTTI STUFFED WITH ZUCCHINI AND TOFU CHEESE

Serves six

2 *tsp. strong or mild cold-pressed olive oil*

½ *onion, finely chopped*

¼ *tsp. marjoram*

1 *tsp. basil*

3 *cloves garlic, chopped*

¼ *green pepper, finely chopped*

6 *mushrooms, coarsely chopped*

2 *small or 1 large zucchini, diced*

2 *T fresh chopped parsley*

1½ *C fresh or canned tomatoes, chopped*

¼ *tsp. pepper*

¼ *tsp. paprika*

salt to taste

½ *lb. firm Chinese tofu, drained and crumbled*

½ *lb. Japanese tofu*

½ *tsp. honey*

1 *clove garlic, sliced and soaked in 2 T olive oil for 45 minutes*

½ *tsp. salt*

dash nutmeg

2 *tsp. lemon juice*

12 to 14 *manicotti shells, cooked al dente (page 166)*

3 *C tomato or pasta sauce*

1. In a large skillet heat the oil. Add the onion, marjoram, and basil. Cook, covered, until the onion is tender. Add the 3 cloves of garlic and cook for 1 minute more. Add the green pepper, mushrooms, and zucchini, toss well, and cook, covered, for 5 minutes. Add the parsley, tomatoes, pepper, paprika, and salt and cook, covered, for 10 minutes. Remove the cover and cook another 5 minutes. There should be no liquid left in the bottom of the skillet.

2. Meanwhile, in a blender or food processor combine the tofu, honey, garlic-olive oil (garlic removed and discarded), salt, nutmeg, and lemon juice and blend until smooth. Stir into the vegetables.

3. Preheat the oven to 350°F. Gently fill each shell with the tofu/vegetable mixture. Lightly cover the bottom of a large baking dish with tomato sauce. Set the manicotti shells side by side in the dish, seam side up, and cover with sauce. Bake, covered, for 20 minutes. Remove the cover and bake 15 minutes more.

Chaya Brasserie's Spaghetti with Japanese Eggplant

Serves six

We got this recipe from Chaya Brasserie, one of the top-rated restaurants in Los Angeles. This Mediterranean dish with a Japanese flair was created by their chef, Shigfumi Tachibe.

½ bell pepper (red, yellow, or green)

1 onion

1 small fennel bulb

5 Japanese eggplants

1 medium zucchini

3 tsp. cold-pressed olive oil

28 oz. can Italian plum tomatoes, or 3½ C chopped fresh tomatoes

6 garlic cloves, minced

½ tsp. ground black pepper

1 tsp. natural soy sauce

1½ lbs. cooked spaghetti

1. Chop the bell pepper, onion, fennel, two of the eggplants, and the zucchini. Heat 1 teaspoon of olive oil in a large skillet, add the chopped vegetables, and cook, covered, until they are just tender. Don't allow them to become mushy.

2. In a medium saucepan, add 1 teaspoon of olive oil, the chopped tomatoes, garlic, and black pepper. Simmer for about 1 hour. Add the cooked vegetables.

3. Preheat the oven to 350°F. Remove the green tops of the remaining eggplants. Cut them lengthwise into ⅛-inch-thick slices. Mix the remaining teaspoon of olive oil and the soy sauce and whisk until completely blended. Brush both sides of each slice with oil–soy sauce mixture. Place them side by side on a thin baking sheet and bake for 5 minutes.

4. If the sauce has cooled, reheat it. Add the cooked spaghetti and some more garlic and pepper if desired. Toss until the spaghetti and the sauce are well mixed. Top each serving with several slices of baked Japanese eggplant and serve.

Pasta e Fagioli

Serves four to five

This recipe is Los Angeles chef Daniel La Bella's favorite and easiest for pasta and beans.

½ lb. dried white beans

4 C Vegetable Stock (page 110) or water with 2 tsp. natural soy sauce

2 tsp. cold-pressed olive oil

2 cloves garlic, chopped

½ onion, finely chopped

¾ C Tomato Sauce (page 163) (canned tomatoes can be used and blended until smooth)

⅛ tsp. basil

⅛ tsp. ground black pepper

½ tsp. paprika

salt to taste

⅛ tsp. cayenne pepper

pinch of thyme

½ celery stalk, sliced ⅛ inch thick

1 small carrot, chopped

⅓ lb. small pasta or spaghetti broken into 2-inch pieces

1. Boil the beans in the broth or seasoned water for 3 minutes. Let them stand for 1½ hours.

2. In a 3-quart saucepan, heat the olive oil and sauté the garlic and onion until lightly golden. Add the Tomato Sauce, basil, black pepper, paprika, salt, cayenne pepper, and thyme. Bring to a boil and simmer for 10 minutes.

3. Combine this sauce with the celery, carrots, and beans in their soaking liquid and simmer for 2 hours or until the beans are tender. Adjust the seasoning.

4. Pass half of the beans through a potato ricer or sieve and return to the beans in the pot.

5. Cook the pasta, drain, and mix with the beans.

PASTA AGLIO E OLIO

Serves four

This is simply pasta with garlic and oil. It's one of the simplest ways of serving pasta. We have changed it a bit to reduce the fat.

1 *lb. whole wheat spaghetti*
    or *fettucini*

1 *tsp. arrowroot* or *kuzu*

⅓ *C water*

1 *T mild cold-pressed olive*
    oil

1 *tsp. strong cold-pressed*
    olive oil

4 *large cloves garlic,*
    chopped

½ *tsp. salt*

1. Cook the pasta according to the package directions.

2. While the pasta is cooking, dissolve the arrowroot in a small amount of water and add to the rest of the water in a small saucepan. Bring to a boil, reduce heat, and simmer for 1 minute, stirring briskly. The mixture will become thick and transparent. Let cool, uncovered, for 15 minutes.

3. Heat the olive oils in a small skillet, add the garlic, and cook until fragrant, about 2 minutes. Transfer the garlic-and-olive-oil mixture to a blender. Add the arrowroot mixture and the salt and blend until creamy.

4. Drain the pasta well. Return to the pot in which it was cooked, mix with the olive oil sauce, and toss well. Serve immediately.

PASTA AL PESTO DI AVOCADO

Serves six

Died-in-the-wool pesto makers pound the garlic, basil, and pine nuts into a paste with a mortar and pestle. However, feel free to use a garlic press to crush the garlic and a mini–food processor or blender to crush the nuts. The basil may be very finely chopped. We don't recommend the use of a blender to purée the avocados because overworking this oily fruit can result in an unpleasant flavor. And remember, the amount of garlic you use is only limited by your taste and your social obligations. This dish is fairly high in fat, so serve it with other dishes containing little or no fat.

3 *cloves garlic, pressed*

¼ *C pine nuts, pulverized in a blender*

15 *large fresh basil leaves, very finely chopped*

¼ *tsp. salt*

½ *tsp. strong cold-pressed olive oil*

1 *large avocado (ripe but not dark), pitted and peeled*

2 *tsp. fresh lemon juice*

water

1 *lb. pasta, cooked according to package directions, or fresh pasta (page 164)*

1. Mix together the pressed garlic, pine nuts, basil, salt, and oil.

2. Mash the avocado with a fork, then pass it through a sieve to make it very creamy. Add the lemon juice, the pine-nut-and-basil mixture, and just enough water to give the pesto the consistency of a thick sauce.

3. The pasta should be quickly drained, slightly wet, and hot. Place the pasta in a heated bowl, cover with the pesto, toss, and serve.

EASY PITA PIZZA

Makes 6 pizzas

This recipe is a lifesaver when you need a great meal or snack, fast. For kids, try adding lightly steamed vegetables that they might otherwise turn down. These pizzas are a treat in lunch boxes.

½ *onion, thinly sliced*

1 *tsp. cold-pressed olive oil*

1 *green pepper, membranes and seeds removed, thinly sliced*

¾ *C Tomato Garbanzo Bean Sauce (page 164) or Tomato Sauce (page 163)*

6 *whole wheat pita breads*

1. Sauté the onion in the olive oil over medium heat for 5 minutes. Remove from the pan. In the same pan, cook the pepper, covered, for 5 minutes over medium heat.

2. To assemble the pizzas, spread 2 tablespoons of the tomato sauce on each pita. Evenly distribute the onions and peppers.

3. Bake at 350°F for 12 to 15 minutes.

VARIATIONS. You can add New Age Italian Sausage (page 155), sautéed mushrooms, sautéed zucchini slices, sliced black olives, or steamed small broccoli florets.

PIZZA DOUGH

Makes 1 12-inch pizza

This classic pizza dough is made with whole wheat flour.

1 *garlic clove, finely sliced*

1 *T cold-pressed olive oil (A strongly scented oil does well here.)*

¾ *C warm water*

1 *package active dry yeast*

dab of honey

1 *T cold-pressed olive oil*

1¼ *C whole wheat flour*

½ *C whole wheat pastry flour*

½ *tsp. salt*

corn meal

1. Soak the garlic in 1 tablespoon of olive oil while you prepare the dough. It will be used to brush on the finished dough before baking.

2. In a large bowl, mix the warm water and yeast. Add the honey and stir to dissolve. Add 1 tablespoon of olive oil (not the oil with the garlic in it) and mix again.

3. Mix the flours and salt and whisk to aerate. Slowly add the flour to the yeast mixture, stirring well with a spoon. Roll the dough into a ball, turn out onto a lightly floured board, cover with a towel, and let stand for 10 minutes in a warm area.

4. Knead the dough for about 10 minutes. It will start out a little sticky but will become smooth and pliable. Form into a ball and place in a large oiled bowl, smooth side down. Roll it over to oil completely, cover with a damp towel, and let it rise in a warm place (about 80°F) for 45 minutes.

5. Preheat the oven to 450°F. Give the dough a light dusting with corn meal. Put it in a 12-inch oiled pizza pan and gently push and press it into place, making a raised lip all around.

6. Brush the dough with the garlic oil to prevent it from becoming soggy after the topping is added. Use only as much as necessary to cover the dough lightly.

7. Cover with your favorite topping and bake for 20 minutes or until the crust starts to brown.

EGGPLANT AND TOMATO PIZZA

Covers 1 12-inch pizza

1 *medium eggplant, washed and dried*

2 *tsp. cold-pressed olive oil*

2 *cloves garlic, chopped*

1 *T salt*

1½ *C chopped fresh* or *canned tomatoes, liquid removed and reserved*

1 *T basil*

¼ *tsp. ground black pepper*

1 *T cold-pressed olive oil*

1 *T soy sauce*

¼ *tsp. garlic powder*

1. Starting at the fattest part of the eggplant, cut seven slices, about ⅕ inch thick. Peel the slices and reserve.

2. Cut the remainder of the unpeeled eggplant into ½-inch cubes.

3. In a large skillet, heat 2 tablespoons of olive oil, add the garlic, and cook for 1 minute. Add the cubed eggplant and salt and cook, covered, for 2 minutes. Add the tomatoes, basil, and pepper and cook, uncovered, for 20 minutes. If the sauce starts to dry out, add some of the tomato liquid. The sauce should be thick.

4. While the eggplant and tomatoes are cooking, mix 1 tablespoon of olive oil, soy sauce, and garlic powder and whisk until the mixture is creamy. Lay the eggplant slices on a lightly oiled baking sheet and brush with the soy sauce mixture.

5. Preheat the broiler. Broil the slices about 5 inches from the heat for 5 to 8 minutes or until the eggplant starts to brown. Carefully turn the slices over, brush with the soy sauce mixture, and cook until lightly browned and tender but not mushy. Use only as much soy sauce mixture as necessary to coat the slices lightly.

6. Preheat the oven to 450°F. Spread the tomato-eggplant mixture over the prepared Pizza Dough (page 181). Place the broiled eggplant on top, overlapping the slices to form a circle on top of the pizza. Bake for 20 minutes or until the crust starts to brown.

BELL PEPPERS STUFFED WITH WALNUT RICE

Serves four

This attractive dish can be made with any sweet peppers: red, green, yellow, and even the lovely purple bell peppers that have recently appeared on produce shelves. Better yet, mix the colors and serve them on a platter garnished with parsley.

4 *bell peppers*

1 *tsp. cold-pressed olive oil*

½ *onion, finely chopped*

¼ *tsp. oregano*

2 *garlic cloves, chopped*

4 *large mushrooms, coarsely chopped*

2 *T chopped parsley*

1 *C cooked tomatoes, chopped*

⅛ *tsp. pepper*

¼ *tsp. salt*

2 *C cooked long-grain brown rice*

½ *C chopped walnuts*

1. Cut off the tops of the peppers on the stem side. The tops should fit back on like a hat. With a paring knife and a spoon, remove the seeds and membranes. Do not pierce the skin. Steam for 4 minutes, then let cool.

2. In a skillet, heat the oil. Add the onion and oregano and cook until the onion is golden. Add the garlic and cook for 1 minute. Add the mushrooms and cook for 5 minutes. Add the parsley, tomatoes, pepper, salt, and rice and cook, covered, for 15 minutes. Add the walnuts and mix well.

3. Preheat the oven to 350°F. Fill each pepper with the rice mixture. Replace the "hats," and bake for 30 minutes.

DINNER CREPES WITH MUSHROOM AND WALNUT FILLING

Makes 9 crepes

THE SAUCE

1 T cold-pressed vegetable oil

1 T whole wheat pastry flour

1 C mild soy milk, hot

1½ C Tomato Sauce (page 163)

THE FILLING

2 tsp. cold-pressed vegetable oil

¾ lb. mushrooms, coarsely chopped

2 cloves garlic, crushed

¼ tsp. thyme

¼ tsp. basil

¼ tsp. salt

⅛ tsp. pepper

¾ C chopped walnuts

THE CREPES

¾ C whole wheat pastry flour

¼ tsp. salt

2 tsp. cold-pressed vegetable oil

1¼ C mild soy milk

1. To prepare the sauce, heat 1 tablespoon of oil in a small saucepan, add the flour and whisk while cooking for 1 minute. Remove from the heat and pour in the hot soy milk all at once. Whisk briskly and return to the heat. Bring to a boil, continuing to whisk, and cook for 2 minutes more or until the sauce has thickened. If lumps appear during cooking, beat with an eggbeater until smooth. Remove ¼ cup of this white sauce and reserve for use in the filling. Combine the rest of the white sauce with the Tomato Sauce and reheat just before serving.

2. To prepare the filling, heat 2 tablespoons of oil in a large skillet and add the mushrooms, garlic, thyme, basil, salt, and pepper. Mix well, cover, and cook for 10 minutes. Remove the cover, add the walnuts, and cook a few minutes more to absorb the extra liquid. Combine with the reserved white sauce.

3. Prepare the crepes last. Sift together the flour and salt. Combine 2 tablespoons of oil and soy milk and mix well. Pour the soy milk mixture into the flour and mix well. If there are small lumps, beat with an egg-

beater for 30 seconds, not more. Heat an 8-inch, nonstick, coated skillet, or coat an uncoated skillet with a thin film of lecithin. When a drop of water sizzles on the skillet, the skillet is ready to cook the crepes. Pour a couple of tablespoons of the batter into the skillet, immediately tipping the skillet around in all directions to coat the bottom completely. Cook for about 1 minute or until the crepe is golden brown.

Loosen the edges of the crepe from the skillet and turn over with a spatula. Cook for another minute. Repeat until all the batter is used up. Stack the crepes on a dish until ready to use.

4. Lay a row of filling down the center of each crepe and roll up. Place them side by side in a serving dish, cover with warm sauce, and serve.

RISOTTO WITH TOMATOES AND GARBANZO BEANS

Serves six

2 C vegetable broth or *water*

½ C white wine, or ⅓ C water, 1 T apple juice, and 1 T white vinegar

1 C long-grain brown rice

2 C Tomato Garbanzo Bean Sauce, chunky (page 164)

1. Bring the broth and wine to a boil and very slowly add the brown rice so that the water continues to boil. Turn down the heat, cover, and cook for 45 to 50 minutes.

2. If by the time the rice is tender the liquid is not completely absorbed, uncover, raise the heat, and cook a few minutes more.

3. Fluff with a fork, add hot Tomato Garbanzo Bean Sauce, and serve.

SUSHI
(NORI MAKI)

Makes 2 rolls

Sushi is a traditional Japanese finger food. The rice used is short-grain and the filling can be almost anything. Both are rolled up in nori, a sea vegetable flattened into a thin sheet. One sheet of nori will produce a roll that can be cut into eight bite-size pieces. Blanched or raw vegetables cut into thin, long strips are ideal. Some suggestions are carrots, string beans, broccoli, green onion, and any color bell pepper. Raw vegetables such as cucumber, jicama, and daikon (Japanese radish) also work well. Use one filling or up to three, and varied colors will make the finished pieces more beautiful. Nori Maki is traditionally rolled with the aid of a bamboo mat made for this purpose (and found at any Japanese food store). However, since most American kitchens lack this utensil, we have found that a clean nonterry kitchen or hand towel also gets the job done.

1 C short-grain brown rice

2½ C cold water

nori sheets

2 T rice vinegar combined with 2 T water in a small dish

vegetables cut into thin strips, ⅛ to ¼ inch thick

SAUCE FOR DIPPING

¼ C natural soy sauce

½ tsp. honey

1 T white vinegar

1 T water

1. To cook the rice, place washed rice and water in a saucepan. Boil, uncovered, for several minutes, cover, reduce heat, and cook for 40 to 50 minutes. The finished rice will be slightly chewy and sticky. Uncover the rice, stir it, and let it stand until it has cooled.

2. On a cutting board or counter lay out the bamboo mat (or towel, narrow end closest to you). Lay a sheet of nori on top of it. Moisten your hands in the vinegar water. Scoop out a small handful of rice and press it onto the nori, making a layer about ½ inch thick. Bring the rice to the edge on three sides. Leave a margin about ¾ inch wide on the edge farthest from you, to seal the finished roll. Lay the vegetables in

straight rows (one row for each vegetable) in the center of the sheet, parallel to the sealing edge. Take the end of the mat or towel closest to you and gently, but firmly, roll it up. Moisten the far edge with vinegar water to seal. With a very sharp knife, slice across the roll, cutting it into eight pieces.

3. Combine all sauce ingredients and dip each piece of sushi before eating.

TACOS

Makes 10 tacos

½ lb. Marinated Tofu (page 142), marinated for no longer than 24 hours

½ lb. Marinated Tempeh (page 141), marinated for no longer than 24 hours

1 tsp. cold-pressed vegetable oil

1 medium onion, finely chopped

2 T tomato paste

½ tsp. chile powder

¼ tsp. ground cumin seed

3 T water

10 taco shells (packaged or baked; page 188)

1 C Guacamole (page 55)

1 large tomato, sliced

shredded lettuce

1 C Salsa (page 53)

1. Remove the tofu and tempeh from the marinade, let them drain in a colander for 20 minutes, then blot to remove any excess marinade.

2. Heat the oil in a skillet and sauté the onion until golden brown. Add the tomato paste, chile powder, cumin seed, and water, and cook, covered, for 5 minutes. Add more water if the ingredients start to stick to the bottom of the pan.

3. Crumble the tofu and tempeh, add them to the filling, and cook, covered for 15 minutes. The sauce should be thick, not runny.

4. Heat the taco shells in the oven at 350°F for 5 minutes. On each shell, place about 2 tablespoons of the filling, 2 tablespoons guacamole, 2 slices tomato, shredded lettuce, and cover with salsa.

NOTE. Use Mexican Black-Eyed Peas (page 225) as a tasty alternative to the tofu filling, especially if they are left over. They are high in fiber and low in fat.

BAKED TACO SHELLS

Packaged taco shells are deep-fried and, therefore, high in saturated fat. You can make your own baked shells that have just a fraction of the fat. It is important that the tortillas be fresh or just thawed. If the tortillas are too dry they will break when you try to fold them.

Corn tortillas

1. If the tortillas are dry, moisten them with a little water, stack them on a plate, cover with waxed paper, and let them stand for 1 hour.

2. Heat the oven to 350°F. Fold the tortillas over without creasing them. Bake for 10 minutes or less. The tortillas should not darken.

BURRITOS

Makes 6 burritos

1 *green pepper, membranes and seeds removed, cut in strips*

1 *tsp. cold-pressed olive oil*

¾ *C cooked brown rice*

1 *ear of corn, cooked, kernels removed*

½ *C canned tomatoes, chopped*

6 *whole wheat tortillas, warmed*

1 *C Mexican Black-Eyed Peas (page 225)*

1 *C Salsa (page 53)*

1 *C Guacamole (page 55)*

sliced black olives

1. Sauté the green pepper in the olive oil over medium heat until tender.

2. In a saucepan, mix the rice, corn, and tomatoes and heat.

3. On each warm tortilla place 4 tablespoons black-eyed peas, 4 tablespoons rice, and several strips of green pepper. Cover with salsa and roll up, folding over the ends. Spoon

3 tablespoons of guacamole over the burrito and top with black olive slices. Serve with Taco Salad (page 120).

NOTE: For Simple Burritos, reheat 1 recipe of A Bowl of Beans (page 223), stirring and mashing until moisture evaporates. Heat tortillas, add a layer of beans, cover with a layer of rice, add Braggs Aminos and cayenne, and roll up as directed in the recipe for Burritos.

TAMALE LASAGNA

Serves four

1 *tsp. cold-pressed olive oil*

1 *onion, chopped*

2 *cloves garlic, chopped*

2 *green peppers, membranes and seeds removed, chopped*

3 *C cooked or canned tomatoes, chopped*

¼ *C water*

½ *tsp. cumin*

½ *tsp. salt*

¼ *tsp. oregano*

¼ *tsp. tarragon*

⅛ *tsp. chile powder*

2 *C fresh corn (two ears)*

12 *corn tortillas*

1. Heat the oil in a large skillet. Sauté the onion and garlic over medium heat until the onion is translucent. Add the green peppers, tomatoes, water, and seasonings. Cook, covered, over medium heat for 10 minutes. Add the corn and continue cooking for 15 minutes more, stirring several times.

2. In the meantime, trim the tortillas to fit into a 9-by-5-inch loaf pan.

3. Preheat the oven to 350°F. Spread a few tablespoons of the to-mato mixture on the bottom of the loaf pan. Place 4 of the trimmed tortillas in a layer over the tomato mixture. Cover the tortillas with approximately one-third of the tomato mixture. Repeat the layering procedure with the remaining tomato mixture.

4. Cover with foil and bake for 1 hour. Serve with a Taco Salad (page 120) or mixed greens.

BAKED RICE AND
GARBANZO BEANS

Serves four

Make this casserole in the morning or the day before and bake it when you need it.

½ *onion, chopped*

1 *tsp. cold-pressed olive oil*

2 *garlic cloves, chopped*

2½ *C cooked long-grain brown rice*

¾ *C cooked or canned garbanzo beans*

½ *C sliced black olives*

1 *T natural soy sauce*

1 *T nutritional yeast*

⅛ *tsp. ground black pepper*

¼ *tsp. paprika*

¼ *tsp. dried basil*

¼ *tsp. dried oregano*

1. Preheat the oven to 350°F. In a skillet, sauté the onion in the olive oil until golden. Add the garlic and cook for 1 minute.

2. Mix all the ingredients well in a large mixing bowl and place in a lightly oiled casserole dish. Bake for 35 minutes. Serve with a green salad and lightly steamed greens or vegetables.

RICE WITH SPRINGTIME VEGETABLES

Serves four

1 tsp. cold-pressed olive oil

3 scallions, chopped

½ C fresh green beans or snow peas, cut into 1-inch pieces

3 ears fresh corn, kernels cut from the cob

1½ C cooked long-grain brown rice

2 T Braggs Aminos sauce or mild soy sauce

Tamari Cashews (page 55)

Heat the oil in a large skillet or wok. Add the onions and cook, covered, until they are tender. Add the beans or snow peas and cook, covered, for 2 minutes. Add the corn and cook, covered, for 5 minutes. Add the cooked rice and Braggs Aminos and mix well. Garnish with Tamari Cashews.

JAMBALAYA

Serves six to eight

1 tsp. cold-pressed olive oil

1 onion, finely chopped

½ lb. mushrooms, stems included, sliced

2 garlic cloves, finely chopped

1 medium green pepper, membranes and seeds removed, diced

1 celery stalk, finely chopped

2½ C fresh or canned tomatoes, chopped

1 C raw long-grain brown rice

2 C water

½ tsp. thyme

2 T finely chopped fresh parsley

¼ tsp. chile powder

½ tsp. paprika

2 T natural soy sauce

¼ tsp. pepper

⅛ tsp. cayenne (optional)

1. Heat the oil in a large skillet. Add the onion and cook, covered, until golden. Add the mushrooms and cook, covered for 5 minutes. Add the garlic, green pepper, and celery and cook, covered, until the pepper is tender.

2. Preheat the oven to 350°F. Add all the remaining ingredients, mixing well to distribute the rice evenly.

3. Place the mixture in a lightly oiled casserole. Cover and bake for 2 hours or until the rice is cooked. Serve with fresh steamed corn and Spinach and Mushroom Salad (page 118).

STEAMED BROWN RICE

Makes 2½ cups

The age of the rice has a lot to do with how much water will be needed to cook it—the older the rice, the more water it will take. Use short-grain brown rice, which tends to be sticky, for stuffings, loaves, and molds. Use long-grain brown whenever you want fluffy rice.

salt
2½ to 3 *C water*

1 *C long-* or *short-grain brown rice*

1. Bring lightly salted water to a fast boil. Gradually pour the rice into the water. When the boiling has resumed, cover the pan. Cook over moderate heat for 45 to 50 minutes.

2. If there is water left in the pot near the end of the cooking time, remove the cover and cook for 5 minutes. If the rice becomes dry too quickly, add ¼ cup boiling water.

RICE PILAF

Serves six

In the Western world, pilaf is usually served as a side dish, accompanying a hunk of meat or poultry. In the Middle East, where it was born, it shares the spotlight with the other main courses.

5 *C broth, or vegetable
   stock, or water*
2 *C long-grain brown rice*
2 *T apple juice*
½ *C unsulfured raisins*
1 *tsp. cold-pressed olive oil*

1 *onion, finely chopped*
4 *small garlic cloves, finely
   chopped*
½ *C slivered almonds*
4 *T chopped parsley*
salt to taste

1. Boil the broth in a large pot. Add the rice slowly to maintain boiling. Reduce the heat and simmer, covered, for 45 minutes. If water remains in the pot after 40 minutes, remove the lid and cook, uncovered, for the last 5 minutes. Add a little boiling water if the rice becomes too dry before it is completely cooked.

2. Place the apple juice and raisins in a small saucepan and bring to a boil. Cook, covered, for 1 minute. Let the raisins stand, covered, for 30 minutes.

3. Heat the oil in a skillet. Add the onion and cook until golden brown. Add the garlic and cook for 1 minute. Add the almonds and parsley and cook for 5 minutes.

4. Combine the cooked rice and plumped raisins in the skillet with the onion and stir them well. Add salt to taste. Serve garnished with parsley sprigs.

ROSEMARY BROWN RICE PILAF

Serves four to six

This pleasant rice dish comes to us from Mrs. Gooch's natural foods market in Los Angeles.

6–8 *shitake mushrooms,*
soaked in water to
cover for 30 minutes
1 *T canola or safflower oil*
1 *large onion, chopped*
⅔ *C diced red bell pepper*
2 *T minced fresh rosemary*

2–3 *T natural instant broth*
powder
1½ *C fresh peas*
4 *C cooked brown rice*
1½ *T black sesame seeds*

1. Remove the mushrooms from the water. Squeeze gently with your hands to expel excess water. Cut away the stems and slice.

2. Heat the oil in a wok or skillet. Cook the onion and mushrooms until the onion is soft. Add the bell pepper and rosemary. Stir in the broth powder. Add the peas and cook for 2 minutes. Stir in the rice and sesame seeds and cook until thoroughly heated. Serve with Grilled Tofu with Summer Vegetables (page 148).

PECAN FRIED RICE

Serves four

1 tsp. cold-pressed vegetable oil

2 green onions, chopped

1 garlic clove, chopped

3 medium mushrooms, chopped

1 small, tender celery stalk, sliced

1 medium carrot, finely chopped

¼ C chopped green pepper

¼ C chopped red cabbage

2½ C cooked long-grain brown rice—day-old rice is best

½ C cubed barbecued tofu (optional)

¼ C chopped pecans

2 T natural soy sauce

1 tsp. toasted sesame seeds

½ tsp. toasted sesame oil

1. Heat the oil in a large skillet. Add half of the green onions, the garlic, mushrooms, celery, carrot, green pepper, and cabbage and stir well. Cook, covered, for 3 minutes.

2. Add the cooked brown rice, tofu, pecans, soy sauce, sesame seeds, and sesame oil and cook, stirring, until the rice is fully heated. Add the remaining green onion and cook for 3 minutes more.

NOTE. Children often don't like the taste of green peppers and toasted sesame oil, so omit these ingredients if the fried rice is to be used in finger pie lunches.

VEGETABLE FRIED RICE

Serves four

2 tsp. cold-pressed vegetable oil

3 cloves garlic, crushed

2 celery stalks, diced

3 medium carrots, diced

3 medium zucchini, sliced

2 C cooked long-grain
  brown rice

2 T natural soy sauce

1. Heat 1 teaspoon of the oil in a large skillet or wok. Add the garlic, celery, and carrots and cook, covered, for 10 minutes over low-medium heat. Add the zucchini and sauté until it is tender but still crisp.

2. Turn up the heat. Wait a few seconds and add 1 teaspoon of the oil. Stir gently and add the rice. Continue stirring while adding the soy sauce. You may vary the amount of soy sauce, according to your taste. Also, feel free to use other spices such as curry or cayenne pepper, and if you like the taste of toasted sesame oil, substitute it for the vegetable oil.

THANKSGIVING PUMPKIN STUFFED WITH RICE AND CHESTNUTS

The question is, of course, "If you don't have turkey on Thanksgiving, what do you have?" The answer is Thanksgiving Stuffed Pumpkin, served whole on a large platter, garnished with parsley, raw cranberries, and orange slices.

1 *medium pumpkin (12 to 14 inches in diameter)*

2 *T honey*

2 *T natural soy sauce*

1 *C water*

½ *lb. fresh chestnuts*

¼ *C unsulfured raisins*

1 *medium red apple, chopped*

½ *C coarsely chopped walnuts*

¼ *C diced celery*

1 *medium onion, chopped*

2 *ears of corn, kernels cut from the cob*

1 *medium green pepper, chopped*

4 *C cooked brown rice*

2 *tsp. cold-pressed vegetable oil*

1 *lb. firm Chinese tofu, diced and drained*

paprika

¼ *tsp. mace*

3 *T Braggs Aminos or mild soy sauce*

¼ *tsp. cinnamon*

parsley sprigs to garnish

1. Preheat the oven to 350°F. Wash the pumpkin and cut off the top. With a large spoon scoop out all of the seeds and strings. Mix the honey and the soy sauce and spread it evenly over the inside of the pumpkin. Place 1 cup water in the bottom of a large baking pan. Put the top back on the pumpkin, place the pumpkin in the baking dish, and cover with foil. Bake for 20 minutes or until the pumpkin is just starting to become tender.

2. Meanwhile, prepare the chestnuts by cutting off the shells using a sharp knife. The chestnuts will have a soft brown skin under the shell. Steam the chestnuts for about 15 minutes, or until they are tender. Rinse them in cool water and slip off

the brown skins. Chop them coarsely.

3. Combine the chestnuts with the raisins, apple, walnuts, celery, onion, corn, green pepper, and brown rice and mix well.

4. Heat the oil in a medium skillet. Add the tofu and enough paprika to give it a pleasing color and cook over high heat for 3 minutes, stirring constantly. Combine the tofu with the rice mixture, mace, Braggs Aminos, and cinnamon and mix until well blended.

5. Fill the pumpkin with this mixture and replace the top. Place it in the baking pan with ¼ inch of water in the bottom. Bake for 45 minutes, garnish with parsley sprigs, and serve.

COUSCOUS WITH TOMATO-EGGPLANT SAUCE

Serves six

1 tsp. cold-pressed olive oil

1 medium onion, chopped

2 large garlic cloves, chopped

1 eggplant, unpeeled, cut into ½-inch cubes

1 green pepper, finely sliced

2 C fresh or canned tomatoes, chopped

½ tsp. salt

½ tsp. pepper

¼ tsp. paprika

¼ tsp. rosemary

4 T finely chopped parsley

¼ tsp. oregano

¼ tsp. basil

1 C water

1 lb. whole wheat couscous, cooked according to package directions

1. Heat the oil in a large skillet. Add the onion and sauté until golden. Add the garlic and cook for 1 minute. Add the eggplant and green pepper and cook for 10 minutes. Add the tomatoes, salt, pepper, paprika, rosemary, parsley, oregano, basil, and water.

2. Cook, covered, for 30 minutes. Stir often to prevent sticking. Mash the eggplant with a fork or hand masher and cook, covered, for 30 minutes more. Serve over cooked couscous.

Tomatoes Stuffed
with Couscous

Serves four

4 *firm medium tomatoes*

¾ *C water*

¼ *tsp. salt*

2 *tsp. cold-pressed olive oil*

½ *C whole wheat couscous*

½ *onion, chopped*

2 *garlic cloves, chopped*

4 *medium mushrooms,
    chopped*

¼ *C chopped almonds*

2 *parsley sprigs, chopped*

salt

pepper

4 *parsley sprigs to garnish*

1. Wash the tomatoes. Cut off the tops and set aside. With a spoon, scoop out the seeds and liquid and reserve. Just before stuffing, gently blot the insides with a paper towel.

2. In a saucepan, bring the water, salt, and 1 teaspoon of the oil to a boil. Add the couscous and bring to a boil. Lower the heat, cover, and cook for 5 minutes, until all the water is absorbed.

3. In a skillet, heat 1 teaspoon of oil, add the onion, and cook until golden brown. Add the garlic and cook 1 minute more. Add the mushrooms, salt lightly, and cook for 3 minutes. Mix with the couscous, almonds, chopped parsley, reserved seeds and liquid, and salt and pepper to taste.

4. Preheat the oven to 350°F. Stuff each tomato with one quarter of the mixture. Put the tomato tops back on and bake for 20 minutes. Garnish with a sprig of parsley.

12

VEGETABLES AND BEANS

ITALIAN-STYLE GREEN BEANS

Serves six

1 *clove garlic, sliced*

2 *tsp. cold-pressed olive oil*

1 *lb. fresh green beans*

2 *T chopped, cooked pimentos*

1 *T pine nuts*

Salt and pepper to taste

1. Soak the garlic in the olive oil for 30 minutes. Remove the garlic and discard and set the oil aside.

2. Wash the beans, remove the ends and strings, and break into 2-inch sections. Steam until just tender, but still crisp. Drain the water and reserve for use in soup or stock. Combine the beans and oil with the remaining ingredients in a saucepan and heat for a few seconds. Serve immediately.

GREEN BEANS WITH ONION AND TOMATOES

Serves six

2 *tsp. cold-pressed olive oil*

1 *medium onion, quartered and thinly sliced*

salt

1 *clove garlic, chopped*

1 *lb. fresh green beans, ends and strings removed and broken into 2-inch pieces*

1 *large tomato, peeled and cut into 12 wedges*

pepper

1. In a large skillet or wok heat the oil, then add the onion. Reduce the heat and sprinkle lightly with salt. Cover and cook slowly until the onion is limp. Add the garlic and cook for 1 minute more.

2. Add the green beans, tomato (including any tomato juices), and pepper to taste. Sprinkle lightly with salt, cover, and cook slowly until the green beans are just tender. Slow, covered cooking will allow the vegetables to stew in their own juices. If the heat is too high, the juices will dry up and the beans will burn. If there is too much juice in the pan when the beans are almost cooked, remove the cover and cook just long enough for the liquid to evaporate. Serve immediately.

BEETS WITH WATERCRESS
AND FRESH DILL

Serves six

Beets generally appear at the dinner table either in the form of soup or in a salad. In this recipe the beets are cooked as a vegetable. The distinct tastes of the three main ingredients blend in a tasty and interesting way.

2 *lb. beets*

1 *tsp. cold-pressed olive oil*

1 *garlic clove, chopped*

1 *bunch watercress, washed, stems removed, cut into 1-inch sections*

1 *sprig fresh dill, chopped (about 1 T)*

¼ *tsp. salt*

1 *T fresh lemon juice*

1. Cut the green tails and all but 1 inch of the stems off the beets. Reserve the greens for use in soup or salad. Steam the whole beets for about 1 hour or until they are tender. The cooking time will vary according to the size of the beets. Rinse them in cold water to cool. Cut off the stems and roots, slip off the peels, and cut into ¼-inch slices. If the beets are large, cut them in half before slicing. Set aside.

2. Heat the oil in a skillet, add the garlic, and cook until fragrant, 1 or 2 minutes. Add the watercress and dill, sprinkle with salt, cover, and cook until the watercress is wilted.

3. Add the sliced beets and lemon juice and toss well.

BROCCOLI AND JAPANESE MUSHROOMS WITH ALMONDS

Serves six

14 *dry shitake mushrooms*
1½ *C water*
1½ *lb. fresh broccoli*
1 *tsp. cold-pressed olive oil*
2 *garlic cloves, finely sliced*
2 *tsp. very finely chopped fresh ginger*

1 *small tomato, chopped*
2 *T slivered almonds*

SAUCE

1 *T arrowroot or kuzu*
3 *T water*
1½ *T soy sauce*

1. Soak the mushrooms in 1½ cups water for 20 minutes.

2. Wash the broccoli. Cut off the stalks, then cut the broccoli into bite-size florets. Peel the stalks, cut into sections 1 inch long, and cut each section lengthwise into thin slices, about ⅛ inch thick. Drain the mushrooms and reserve the water. Remove the stems, discard, and cut the mushrooms into strips.

3. Heat the oil in a wok or large skillet. Add the garlic and ginger and cook until the garlic is fragrant, about 2 minutes. Add the mushrooms, broccoli, and tomato and cook for 5 minutes. Add enough water to the mushroom water to make 1½ cups and add to the broccoli. Cook until the broccoli is tender, about 10 minutes more.

4. Prepare the sauce while the broccoli is cooking by dissolving the arrowroot in 3 tablespoons of water. Add the soy sauce.

5. When the broccoli is tender, add the sauce and the almonds and stir constantly, until the sauce is thickened. Add more soy sauce to taste. Serve over a bed of long-grain brown rice with a Chinese Green Salad (page 116).

ITALIAN-STYLE BROCCOLI

Serves four to six

1 *clove garlic, sliced*

2 *tsp. cold-pressed olive oil*

1 *bunch broccoli*

salt and pepper to taste

1. Soak the garlic in the olive oil for 20 minutes. Remove the garlic and discard.

2. Steam the broccoli until it is just tender and a bright green color. Pour off the water and reserve for use in a soup. Remove the steaming rack and put the broccoli into the saucepan. Add the garlic oil, salt, and pepper and toss gently until all the pieces are coated. Heat for several seconds. Serve immediately.

BROCCOLI WITH GARLIC AND CAPERS

Serves four

1 *bunch of broccoli, washed and drained*

1 *tsp. cold-pressed olive oil*

¼ *large onion, thinly sliced*

salt to taste

2 *garlic cloves, finely chopped*

2 *T capers plus liquid*

1. Cut off the stems of the broccoli, peel them, then cut into 1-inch sections, and slice lengthwise. Cut the broccoli tops into bite-size florets.

2. Heat the oil in a large skillet or wok. Add the onions, sprinkle very lightly with salt, cover, and cook until the onions are limp. Do not allow them to brown.

3. Add the garlic and cook for 1 minute. Add the capers along with the caper liquid. Add the broccoli and sprinkle lightly with salt. Cook, covered, at medium heat until the broccoli is tender but still crisp and bright green.

STUFFED CABBAGE

Serves six (about 15 rolls)

Make plenty for leftovers. They keep well in the refrigerator for several days and they're good cold or hot.

SAUCE

1 *tsp. cold-pressed olive oil*

½ *onion, chopped*

juice of ½ *lemon*

28 *oz. cooked or canned*
  tomatoes

1 *C apple juice*

½ *C unsulfured raisins*

⅛ *tsp. thyme*

¼ *tsp. salt*

FILLING

1 *large green cabbage*

1 *tsp. cold-pressed olive oil*

2 *scallions, chopped*

1 *carrot, chopped*

½ *celery stalk, chopped*

1 *mushrooms, halved and*
  sliced

3 *T chopped parsley*

½ *C chopped pistachios*

1 *C unsulfured raisins*

⅛ *tsp. thyme*

1 *T soy sauce*

2 *tsp. vinegar*

1 *T vegetable broth* or *water*

dash of nutmeg

2 *C cooked short-grain*
  brown rice

1. To make the sauce, heat 1 teaspoon of oil in a large skillet. Add the onion and cook until soft. Add the remaining sauce ingredients. Simmer, covered, for 1 hour. Cool a few minutes and purée in a blender. The sauce can be prepared a day in advance if desired.

2. While the sauce is cooking, wash the cabbage and steam in a large pot for 6 minutes. Let cool for a few minutes and remove the softened outer leaves. Do not try to re-move leaves that are still crisp. Put the cabbage back into the pot and steam for 6 minutes more. Let cool and remove the softened leaves. You will need about twenty leaves. The outer leaves will be the largest; those inside will be quite small so you'll have to double those up. Return the separated leaves to the steaming pot and steam for 6 minutes more. With a sharp knife shave down the thick part of the stalk to make folding easier. Set aside. Chop

enough of the leftover cabbage and cabbage parings to make 1 cup.

3. Heat 1 teaspoon of oil in a large skillet. Add the chopped cabbage, scallions, carrot, celery, mushrooms, parsley, pistachios, raisins, and thyme. Cover and cook for 5 minutes. Add the soy sauce, vinegar, broth or water, and nutmeg and cook, covered, for 7 minutes more. Stir in the rice. Set aside.

4. Preheat the oven to 350°F. Cover the bottom of a deep baking dish or casserole with about ¼ inch of sauce. Fill the large leaves first by placing a heaping tablespoon of the rice mixture in the center. Fold up the bottom (shaved stalk), fold over the sides, then fold down the top. Place, seam side down, in a baking dish. Cover with the sauce and another layer of stuffed cabbage. Repeat until you've used up all the leaves. When the leaves become too small to close, place a piece of the smallest leaves over the filling and close. Pour the remaining sauce on top, shaking the dish gently to distribute the sauce. Bake for 1 hour. Serve over a shallow bed of brown rice.

RED CABBAGE
WITH APPLES AND WINE

Serves six

1 *medium red cabbage, thinly sliced*

2 *green apples, coarsely chopped*

1 *onion, chopped*

½ *C white wine*

¼ *C unsulfured raisins*

1 *T vinegar*

1 *T lemon juice*

1 *T molasses*

⅛ *tsp. pepper*

½ *tsp. salt*

¼ *tsp. caraway seeds*

Combine all the ingredients in a saucepan and cook, covered, for 25 minutes.

EGGPLANT PARMIGIANA

Serves four

Los Angeles chef Daniel LaBella says that the secret of this recipe is in the preparation of the eggplant. Leftovers make delicious sandwiches.

SAUCE

2 *cloves garlic, chopped*

2 *T cold-pressed olive oil*

12 *oz. tomato paste*

28 *oz. canned whole* or *crushed tomatoes*

1 *C water*

EGGPLANT CUTLETS

1 *firm eggplant*

salt

2 *C whole wheat bread crumbs*

¼ *tsp. garlic powder*

½ *C mild soy milk*

½ *C whole wheat pastry flour in plastic bag*

1 *T olive oil for cooking*

1. To make the sauce, cook the garlic in 2 tablespoons of olive oil in a large skillet until golden brown. Remove the garlic from the skillet and reserve.

2. Add the tomato paste to the skillet and cook at medium-high heat for 5 minutes, stirring constantly. Add the canned tomatoes and water and break them up. Bring to a fast boil and add the reserved garlic. Reduce the heat, cover, and simmer for 1 hour.

3. To prepare the cutlets, peel the eggplant and slice ⅛ inch thick. Salt each slice lightly and pile the slices in a large colander. Cover with a clean kitchen towel and allow to stand for 2 hours to leach out any bitterness.

4. Mix the bread crumbs, garlic powder, salt, and pepper in a flat-bottom bowl or deep dish. Place the soy milk in a separate bowl.

5. Place the eggplant slices, three at a time, in a plastic bag with the flour and shake. Remove the slices, one at a time, and shake off any excess flour. Dip in the soy milk and dredge in bread crumbs. Repeat with all the eggplant slices.

6. Heat 1 tablespoon olive oil in a large skillet and sauté the eggplant slowly, covered, for about 4 minutes, turn, and cook for 4 minutes

more. Test with fork. The slices should be crispy on the outside and tender on the inside.

7. Preheat the oven to 350°F. To assemble, spread a couple of tablespoons of sauce on the bottom of a lightly oiled baking dish. Lay out a single layer of eggplant and cover with sauce. Repeat to make a double layer. Bake, covered, for 30 minutes.

BARBECUED EGGPLANT

Serves four

1 *eggplant*
Barbecue Sauce (page 135)

salt

1. Preheat the oven to 350°F. Peel and cut the eggplant into ⅓-inch-thick slices. Salt the slices. Place on a rack or colander and let stand for 30 minutes. Wipe off salt with a clean kitchen towel.

2. Lay the slices out on a lightly oiled baking sheet. Brush on barbecue sauce. Bake for 15 minutes. Turn over, brush with barbecue sauce, and bake for 15 minutes more or until the eggplant is tender but not mushy.

MOUSSAKA

Serves four

Traditional moussaka is made with deep-fried eggplant, either beef or lamb, and generous amounts of cheese. This version is much lower in fat but still delicious.

1 *large eggplant*

1 *tsp. salt*

1 *tsp. garlic*

SAUCE

4 *tsp. cold-pressed olive oil*

½ *large onion, finely chopped*

2 *cloves garlic, chopped*

2 *T whole wheat pastry flour*

1 *C mild soy milk*

1 *C cooked or canned tomatoes, chopped*

1 *tsp. paprika*

⅛ *tsp. ground cloves*

⅛ *tsp. nutmeg*

⅛ *tsp. oregano*

⅛ *tsp. basil*

½ *tsp. salt*

RICE FILLING

2 *tsp. cold-pressed olive oil*

¼ *large onion, finely chopped*

¼ *lb. small mushrooms, sliced*

1 *T fresh parsley, finely chopped*

1 *T natural soy sauce*

½ *tsp. dill*

2 *C cooked short-grain brown rice*

CRUMB TOPPING

¼ *C whole wheat bread crumbs*

2 *tsp. cold-pressed olive oil*

1. Remove the stem from the eggplant, then peel and cut into slices ⅓ inch thick. Boil water in a large pot, add the salt, garlic, and eggplant. Cook until the eggplant is tender and has lost its creamy whiteness, about 6 minutes. Drain in a colander while preparing the other ingredients.

2. For the sauce, heat 1 teaspoon of the olive oil in a large skillet. Add

the onion and garlic and cook, covered, until the onion is lightly browned. In a small saucepan heat 3 more teaspoons of the olive oil. Add the flour, and cook 3 minutes over low-medium heat, stirring constantly. Do not allow the flour to brown or scorch as this will impart an unpleasant flavor.

3. Slowly add the soy milk to the flour, mixing quickly with a wire whisk. Add the tomatoes, paprika, cloves, nutmeg, oregano, basil, and salt and bring to a boil, stirring constantly, while the sauce thickens. Cook 2 minutes more.

4. For the rice filling, heat 2 teaspoons of oil in the same large skillet. Add the onion and cook until transparent. Add the mushrooms and cook, covered, for 5 minutes. Add the parsley, soy sauce, and dill and cook, covered, for 3 minutes. Turn off the heat and mix in the brown rice.

5. Preheat the oven to 350°F. Cover the bottom of a casserole dish with a small amount of sauce. Place a single layer of eggplant slices over it. Cover with more sauce. Add half the rice and spread evenly over the sauce. Cover the rice with more sauce and repeat the layers until all the ingredients are used up. Finish with a layer of eggplant, covered with the rest of the sauce. Shake the casserole gently back and forth to settle the layers and allow the sauce to run throughout.

6. Mix the bread crumbs with 2 teaspoons of olive oil. Spread the crumb topping evenly over the top and press it gently in place. Bake for 1 hour.

EGGPLANT FLORENTINE

Serves four to six

1 *medium eggplant*

1 *lb. mushrooms*

1 *T cold-pressed olive oil*

salt to taste

1 *clove garlic, crushed*

4 *bunches spinach*
  (approximately 2 lb.)

1 *tsp. cold-pressed olive oil*

¼ *tsp. garlic powder*

1 *T lemon juice*

4 *T cold-pressed olive oil*

2 *T soy sauce*

¼ *tsp. onion powder*

1. Peel the eggplant and slice ⅓ to ¼ inch thick. Salt each slice lightly. Put a clean kitchen towel on a dinner plate and place the eggplant slices on the towel for 1 hour. In the meantime, prepare the mushrooms and spinach.

2. To prepare the mushrooms, wipe them with a clean dry kitchen towel to clean. Slice. Heat 1 tablespoon of oil in a large skillet, add the mushrooms, salt, and crushed garlic. Sauté until tender, about 7 minutes, stirring often, then remove the mushrooms and reserve.

3. To prepare the spinach, cut off the leaves and save the stems for soup stock. Wash each leaf well. Cut the large leaves into three parts. The small leaves need not be cut. Place the spinach in a skillet, salt lightly, cover, and cook just until the spinach wilts. Uncover, add 1 teaspoon of the olive oil, garlic powder,

and lemon juice, salt to taste, and cook a few minutes more, until the liquid has evaporated.

4. To broil the eggplant, wipe off each slice with a clean kitchen towel. Mix 4 tablespoons of olive oil, the soy sauce, and onion powder and blend well with a wire whisk. Arrange the eggplant slices in a single layer on a lightly oiled baking sheet. Brush each slice with the olive oil mixture. Broil 5 to 6 inches from the heat for about 5 minutes. Turn each slice over, brush with the olive oil mixture, and broil another 5 minutes. Use only as much of the oil–soy sauce mixture as you need to coat each slice lightly on both sides. Test with a fork. The eggplant should be very tender but not mushy.

5. Arrange the eggplant attractively on a bed of spinach and top with the mushrooms.

EGGPLANT AL FORNO

Serves six

2 *medium eggplants*
salt
½ *C soy milk*
1 *C Seasoned Bread
  Crumbs (below)*

3 *T cold-pressed olive oil*
1 *tsp. water*
2 *C Tomato Sauce (page
  163)*
1¾ *C Tofu Cheese (page
  214)*

1. Wash and peel the eggplants. Cut into slices about ⅓ inch thick, and with the tip of a knife, scrape away any excess seeds. Salt the slices and place on a rack or colander for 30 minutes, then dry with a clean kitchen towel. Dip each slice in soy milk and roll in bread crumbs to cover completely.

2. In a large skillet, heat 2 teaspoons of the olive oil. Place the eggplant in a single layer and cook, covered, at medium heat until browned, about 5 minutes. Turn the slices over, sprinkling a few drops of the remaining olive oil beneath each piece. Add a teaspoon of water, cover, and cook until the eggplant is tender but not mushy, about 5 minutes more.

3. Preheat the oven to 350°F. Spread the bottom of the baking dish with a thin layer of tomato sauce. Arrange the eggplant in a single layer over it and cover each slice with a tablespoon of tofu cheese. Add another layer of eggplant, and cover again with tofu cheese. Cover generously with tomato sauce. Bake for 30 minutes.

SEASONED BREAD CRUMBS
(Makes 1 cup)

4 *slices whole wheat bread,
  dried*
1 *tsp. dried basil*
1 *tsp. dried oregano*

½ *tsp. powdered garlic*
½ *tsp. celery seed*
½ *tsp. salt*

1. Break the dried bread into small pieces and place in a blender or food processor with all the other ingredients.

continued on next page

Eggplant al Forno (cont.)

2. Blend at medium speed to make crumbs.

TOFU CHEESE
(Makes 1³/₄ cups)

1 *clove garlic, sliced*

1 *T cold-pressed olive oil*

½ *lb. firm Chinese tofu,*
  drained and crumbled

½ *lb. Japanese tofu, drained*

½ *tsp. honey*

½ *tsp. salt*

dash of nutmeg

1 *T fresh chopped parsley*

2 *tsp. lemon juice*

1. Soak the garlic in the olive oil for 45 minutes, then discard the garlic.

2. Place all the ingredients in a blender or food processor and blend at high speed until creamy.

PAN-COOKED SPINACH

Serves four

2 *bunches spinach*

2 *tsp. cold-pressed olive oil*

½ *onion, finely chopped*

2 *garlic cloves, finely*
  chopped

salt

pepper

1. Wash the spinach well to remove all the sand. Remove the stems and cut the large leaves into two or three pieces. The smaller leaves may be left whole.

2. Heat the oil in a very large skillet. Add the onion and cook, covered, until tender. Add the garlic and cook for 1 minute more. Add the spinach, sprinkle lightly with salt and pepper and cook, covered, until the spinach wilts. Remove the cover and cook a few minutes more until all the liquid evaporates. The spinach should not be overcooked.

PAN-COOKED SUMMER SQUASH

Serves four

1 lb. fresh summer squash
1 tsp. mild cold-pressed
    olive oil

2 large cloves garlic,
    crushed
salt to taste

1. Wash the squash and slice it about ⅕ inch thick.

2. In a large skillet heat the olive oil. Add the squash and stir to coat completely. Add the crushed garlic and salt. Cover and cook over medium heat for 10 minutes. Shake the skillet frequently to avoid burning. The squash will be golden.

Cauliflower Gratinée

Serves six

1 *cauliflower, washed*

1 *T cold-pressed olive oil*

1 *T whole wheat pastry flour*

½ *tsp. mild nutritional yeast*

1 *C mild soy milk, hot*

¼ *tsp. salt*

dash pepper

dash coriander

¼ *tsp. garlic powder*

¼ *tsp. vinegar*

½ *C fresh whole wheat bread crumbs (not dried)*

1 *tsp. cold-pressed olive oil*

1. Break the cauliflower into bite-size florets. Steam for 4 minutes and set aside.

2. In a small saucepan, heat 1 tablespoon of oil, add the flour and nutritional yeast, and stir briskly over medium heat for 1 minute. Remove from the heat and pour in the soy milk, all at once, and whisk. If lumps appear, beat with an eggbeater until smooth. Add the salt, pepper, coriander, garlic powder, and vinegar. Return to the heat and bring to a boil, whisking constantly until the sauce is thickened. Cook for 2 minutes more.

3. Place the cauliflower evenly in an oiled baking dish. Cover evenly with the sauce.

4. Preheat the oven to 350°F.

5. Combine the bread crumbs and 1 teaspoon of oil and mix until the crumbs are well coated. Sprinkle over the cauliflower. Cover with foil and bake for 30 minutes. Uncover and place under the broiler for 2 minutes or until the crumbs are browned.

BROILED POTATO CHIPS

About ½ to 1 medium potato per person

Small to medium white or
red potatoes
1 T cold-pressed olive oil

1 T natural soy sauce
salt to taste

Wash the potatoes and slice them very thinly. Mix the oil and soy sauce and whisk until blended. Brush the slices lightly on both sides with this mixture and lay them in a single layer on a baking sheet so that they do not overlap. Brush lightly with olive oil. Broil at middle level for about 7 minutes or until golden. Turn and broil another 3 to 5 minutes, until golden. The broiling time can vary, so keep a close eye on the chips as they cook. Dark chips will be bitter. Salt to taste, if desired. If made in advance, the chips are easily reheated in the oven.

BOUNTY CUSTARD

Serves four

This makes a delightful holiday vegetable dish, in place of mashed potatoes.

4 C fresh banana squash,
    peeled and cut into
    chunks
3 T natural maple syrup
¼ tsp. salt

3 T raw almond butter or
    raw tahini
½ tsp. natural vanilla
    flavoring

1. Steam the squash until it is soft.

2. Place all the ingredients in a food processor or blender and blend until the mixture is smooth. Serve hot.

VARIATION. To serve as a dessert, stir in ¼ cup broken pecan pieces and chill.

BAKED POTATO

A baked potato is filling, nourishing, and low in fat and calories as long as it's bare. Add the butter and sour cream to make it moist and you'll likely have to pedal to Patagonia to work it off. This recipe is our solution to the moist and low-fat baked potato dilemma.

large, thick-skinned baking potatoes
vegetable broth or *water*

seasonings to taste
olive oil

1. Preheat the oven to 350°F. Wash and dry the potatoes. Puncture the skin once with a fork. Place, puncture side up, on the oven rack and bake for 50 to 60 minutes, depending on the size. When the potatoes are cooked they will yield when pressed.

2. Allow them to cool until they can be handled but are still hot. Cut them in half and carefully scoop out the insides into a bowl. Save the skins. Add enough broth or water to make them moist and mix well. Season to taste with salt and pepper and a dash of garlic powder or any other seasoning you like. Chopped chives or scallions can be mixed in.

3. Fill each skin with prepared potatoes, brush the tops lightly with olive oil, and place 5 inches under the broiler for 5 minutes or until the tops brown lightly.

POTATO STEAKS ALMONDINE

Serves four

2 *baking potatoes*
4 *tsp. cold-pressed olive oil*
1 *T natural soy sauce*
2 *cloves garlic, chopped*

¼ *C sliced almonds*
1 *T water*
1 *T dry white wine*
Salt and pepper to taste

1. Steam the potatoes in their skins until tender when a fork is inserted. Cool for 15 minutes, then slip off the skins. Cool for another 30 minutes.

2. Slice the cooled potatoes lengthwise, ¼ to ⅕ inch thick.

3. Preheat the broiler. Mix 3 teaspoons of the olive oil and the soy sauce and whisk until smooth. Brush both sides of the slices lightly with this mixture (saving any left over to add to the sauce) and lay the slices in a single layer on a baking sheet. Broil for about 7 minutes, or until the potatoes are golden. Turn them and brown the other side, 3 to 5 minutes. All broilers are different, so keep a close watch on the potatoes as they brown so they don't scorch and become bitter.

4. To make the sauce, heat the remaining teaspoon of olive oil in a small pan. Add the garlic and cook for 1 minute, then add the almonds, the rest of the soy sauce–oil mixture used for basting the potatoes, the water, and the wine. Add salt and pepper to taste. Warm up the sauce mixture, just to heat through, then turn off the heat immediately. Serve the potatoes on a bed of cooked spinach or other cooked greens and spoon sauce over the potatoes.

POTATOES MILANESE

Serves four to six

1 *clove garlic, finely sliced*

1 *T plus* 1 *tsp. cold-pressed olive oil*

15 *small new red potatoes*

½ *onion, thinly sliced*

salt to taste

1 *T finely chopped parsley*

1. Soak the garlic in 1 tablespoon of the olive oil for ½ hour. Remove the garlic and discard.

2. Steam the potatoes until tender but not soft. The skins should not break. Let cool for 15 minutes.

3. Sauté the onion in the remaining olive oil for 10 minutes, covered, over medium heat. The onion should be translucent and slightly golden.

4. Slice the potatoes about ¼ inch thick and mix with the onions, garlic oil, and salt. Sprinkle the parsley on top.

POTATOES CONSTANTIN

Serves six to eight

12 *new potatoes*

2 *C canned tomatoes, chopped*

2 *tsp. soy sauce*

1 *tsp. cold-pressed olive oil*

1 *tsp. vinegar*

¼ *tsp. garlic powder*

dash of pepper

1. Preheat the oven to 350°F. Wash the potatoes and slice into thin ovals.

2. Mix the remaining ingredients and combine well with the potatoes. Bake, uncovered, in a casserole dish for 1 hour, or until potatoes are tender.

COUNTRY POTATOES

Serves six

1 *garlic clove*

1 *tsp. cold-pressed olive oil*

8 *new potatoes*

1 *tsp. cold-pressed olive oil*

1 *carrot, diced*

½ *C fresh peas*

1 *T vegetable broth* or *water*

salt to taste

pepper to taste

1. Bruise the garlic clove with a fork and place in 1 teaspoon olive oil. Set aside.

2. Steam the potatoes whole and unpeeled until tender, about 20 minutes.

3. Heat the remaining teaspoon of olive oil in a medium skillet. Add the carrot and peas and cook, covered, for 5 minutes. Add the broth or water and cook, covered, at medium heat until the carrots are just tender, about 7 minutes.

4. When the potatoes are tender, allow them to cool until they can be handled. Slip off the skins, cut in half, and slice. Add to the cooked carrot and peas.

5. Remove the garlic from the olive oil and discard the garlic. Add the garlic oil to the vegetables and mix well but gently. Heat slightly if the potatoes are cool. Adjust the seasoning.

MALIBU CHILE

Serves eight

Although fresh mushrooms can be used in this dish, mushrooms that have been stored in a closed container or plastic bag in the refrigerator for one week impart a hearty flavor to our chile. Serve as a main dish with coleslaw and potato salad, or as a companion to tofu ribs, pecan herb burgers, or tofu hot dogs. Malibu Chile is also good in finger pies, burritos, and pita sandwiches.

1 *tsp. cold-pressed olive oil*

1 *large onion, finely chopped*

4 *cloves garlic, chopped*

4 *small sweet carrots, shredded*

1 *lb. pinto beans, soaked overnight (or covered with boiling water and soaked for 1 hour before cooking)*

¼ *lb. week-old mushrooms, very finely chopped*

6 *oz. can tomato paste*

1 *green pepper, seeds and membranes removed*

6 *C water*

2 *level T chile powder*

2 *level tsp. ground cumin*

2 *tsp. salt*

⅛ *tsp. ground coriander*

½ *tsp. ground celery seeds*

½ *bay leaf*

½ *tsp. basil*

1. Heat the oil in a large pot. Add the onions and cook until golden. Do not scorch.

2. Add the garlic and shredded carrots and cook for 5 minutes longer, stirring often.

3. Add the remaining ingredients and cook, uncovered, over medium heat for 4 hours. Stir regularly to avoid scorching. If the chile becomes too dry, add a little boiling water. At the end of the cooking time, the chile should be thick.

APPLE-HONEY BAKED BEANS

Serves six to eight

1 *lb. pinto or kidney beans, soaked overnight*

5 *C water*

¾ *medium onion, finely sliced*

1 *apple, cored and diced*

½ *C honey*

1 *T olive oil*

1 *tsp. dry mustard*

1 *tsp. ginger powder*

1. Drain the beans. Place in a saucepan with water and cook for 45 minutes or until the beans are just tender. Drain and reserve the liquid.

2. Preheat the oven to 350°F. In a casserole dish mix the beans, onion, and apple. In a separate bowl mix the honey, seasonings, and 2 cups of the bean liquid. If there is not enough bean liquid add fresh water and pour over the beans.

3. Bake, covered, for 3 hours. Stir once and bake 1 hour more, uncovered. If the beans are too dry, add some boiling bean liquid or water. Serve with Carrot Almond Salad (page 121).

A BOWL OF BEANS

Serves six to eight

6½ *C water*

3 *C dried beans (2 C azuki; 1 C pinto), soaked overnight, drained*

3 *large cloves garlic*

3 *T Braggs Aminos or more to taste*

Bring water to a boil and cook beans over low heat for 40 minutes, covered. Add garlic and Braggs Aminos and cook another 30 minutes, or until just tender.

CHILEAN BLACK-EYED PEAS
AND WINTER SQUASH

Serves six

Our friend, Carlos Hagen-Lautrup, is a geographer and curator of maps, but best of all, he's a brilliant chef. In his native Chile, he uses fresh black-eyed peas, harvested ripe off the vine. If you happen to be lucky enough to run across any of these fresh beans, use them; otherwise use the dried, packaged kind.

1 *lb. dried black-eyed peas, soaked overnight, or 2½ C fresh black-eyed peas*

1 *T cold-pressed vegetable oil*

2 *lb. winter squash, diced*

2 *large onions, chopped*

4 *ears of corn, kernels cut off the cob*

2 *large tomatoes, sliced*

1 *small chile (if you like it hot; otherwise use ½ chili), finely chopped*

3 to 6 *cloves garlic, finely chopped*

1 *T paprika*

½ *tsp. salt*

1 *tsp. basil*

1 *T oregano*

3 *bay leaves*

¼ *tsp. whole peppercorns*

½ *tsp. whole cumin seeds*

½ *tsp. coriander seeds, whole*

¼ to ½ *tsp. chile powder*

1. Drain the soaked black-eyed peas. Place them in a large saucepan, cover with water, bring to a boil, and simmer for 20 minutes. They will be half-cooked. Drain and rinse them in cold water. Drain again and set aside.

2. Heat the oil in a large skillet and add the squash, onions, corn, tomatoes, chile, garlic, paprika, and salt. Cook, stirring often, for 10 minutes.

3. Add the cooked vegetables to the black-eyed peas, and add fresh water to cover. Cover the saucepan, and bring the mixture to a boil. Add basil, oregano, bay leaves, peppercorns, cumin seeds, coriander seeds, and chile powder. Reduce the heat and simmer, covered, for about 25

minutes. Taste often to correct the seasoning.

NOTE. Remove the bay leaves as soon as the beans are cooked.

Mexican Black-Eyed Peas

Makes 2½ cups

This dish is usually made with black beans, but we prefer the sweetness and full-bodied flavor of black-eyed peas. It is simple and delicious

1 *C raw black-eyed peas*
3 *C water*
2 *T natural soy sauce*

¼ *tsp. ground cumin*
½ *tsp. chile powder*

1. Either soak the black-eyed peas in water overnight or boil the water, pour it over the peas, and let it stand for 1½ hours.

2. Put the black-eyed peas, soaking water, and all the other ingredients in a saucepan and bring to a boil. Lower heat and cook for 1½ hours or until the beans are very tender. Serve with steamed vegetables or greens and a salad, or in burritos, tacos, or finger pies.

PICCADILLO

Serves six

Piccadillo is traditionally made with leftover meat. We think it's a great dish on its own, so here it is, minus the leftovers.

2 C water

¼ tsp. salt

1 C pinto beans, soaked
    overnight and drained

1 tsp. paprika

⅛ tsp. pepper

1 tsp. cold-pressed olive oil

1 onion, minced

1 sweet pepper (green,
    yellow, or red), chopped

2 fresh tomatoes, chopped

1½ T capers, minced

½ C unsulfured raisins

½ C chopped unsulfured
    dried apricots

⅛ tsp. cayenne (optional)

salt to taste

1 tsp. fresh lemon juice

6 C cooked long-grain
    brown rice

1. Bring the water and salt to a boil. Add the beans, paprika, and pepper and cook for 1½ hours or until the beans are cooked but not mushy. Stir often to keep the beans from sticking. Add a little water if the beans become too dry.

2. Heat the olive oil in a skillet, add the onion, and cook until soft. Add pepper and cook for 5 minutes. Add the tomatoes, capers, raisins, apricots, cayenne, salt, and lemon juice. Cover and cook for 30 minutes. Mix with the beans. Serve on a bed of brown rice.

STUFFED ACORN SQUASH

Serves four

2 acorn squash

¼ tsp. salt

⅛ tsp. pepper

⅛ tsp. cinnamon

1 tsp. cold-pressed olive oil

2 celery stalks, chopped

2 carrots, chopped

6 mushrooms, halved and sliced

4 scallions, sliced

4 T fresh chopped parsley

¼ C chopped almonds

¼ C unsulfured raisins

¼ tsp. pepper

½ tsp. salt

2 T white wine, or 2 T vegetable broth and ½ tsp. vinegar

2 T water

2 T natural soy sauce

1. Cut the squash in half lengthwise. Scoop out seeds and fibers. Mix the salt, pepper, and cinnamon and sprinkle inside and around the rim of the squash. Set aside.

2. Heat the oil in a skillet. Add the celery, carrots, mushrooms, scallions, and parsley and cook, covered, for 5 minutes. Add all the other ingredients to the skillet, except squash, and cook, covered, for 7 minutes. Most of the liquid should be absorbed. If not, remove the cover and cook for 1 minute more.

3. Preheat the oven to 350°F. Put ⅓ inch of water in the bottom of a baking dish. Fill the squash with vegetable mixture, set shell side down in the baking dish, cover with foil, and bake for 40 minutes.

VEGETABLE CURRY

Serves six

2 *C water*

1 *C shredded dried coconut*

1 *tsp. cold-pressed olive oil*

½ *medium onion, quartered and sliced*

4 *garlic cloves, minced*

1 *T fresh grated ginger*

Curry Powder (see ingredients to the right)

2 *T water*

2 *medium tomatoes, very finely chopped*

10 *green beans, cut into 1-inch pieces*

2 *C cubed baking potatoes (about 1 large potato)*

3 *medium carrots, diagonally cut into ½-inch-long pieces*

1 *C red cabbage, diced*

4 *large mushrooms, quartered, or 12 button mushrooms*

½ *tsp. salt*

2 *C cauliflower, cut into small florets (about ½ head)*

1 *small stalk broccoli, cut into florets, stem peeled and sliced*

2 *T fresh lemon juice*

cooked brown rice

cilantro, finely chopped

CURRY POWDER

½ *tsp. dry mustard*

½ *tsp. cinnamon*

2 *tsp. cumin*

2 *tsp. coriander*

1 *tsp. tumeric*

2 *tsp. paprika*

½ *tsp. allspice*

dash cayenne (optional)

¼ *tsp. ground cloves*

1. Boil 2 cups of water and coconut for 1 minute and let stand for 1 hour. Blend at high speed in blender for 3 minutes. Pour through several layers of damp cheesecloth and wring to extract as much liquid as possible; discard the pulp. Two cups of natural unsweetened coconut milk may be used (not the clear liquid found in fresh unripe coconuts).

2. Mix the curry powder ingredients. Heat the oil in a large skillet. Add the onion and cook slowly until golden. Add the garlic and ginger and cook for 2 minutes more. Mix

the curry powder with 2 tablespoons of water to form a paste. Add the tomatoes and curry paste and cook, covered, for 5 minutes. Do not allow the mixture to scorch. Add the green beans, potatoes, carrots, cabbage, mushrooms, salt, and coconut liquid; boil, reduce heat, and cook about 20 minutes or until all vegetables are tender. Add the cauliflower and broccoli and cook until just tender. Turn off the heat and stir in the lemon juice. Serve over cooked brown rice. Garnish with cilantro.

ZUCCHINI WITH GARLIC AND BASIL

Serves four

1 *tsp. cold-pressed olive oil*
2 *cloves garlic, minced*
2 *medium zucchini, sliced*

2 *T fresh chopped basil leaves*
salt to taste
pepper to taste

Heat the oil in a large skillet. Add the garlic and cook for 1 minute. Add the zucchini, basil, salt, and pepper and cook, covered, for 5 minutes. Uncover, and cook until the zucchini is tender but not soft.

MIXED VEGETABLES, JAPANESE STYLE

Serves four

1 *tsp. cold-pressed olive oil*

1 *onion, chopped*

8 *mushrooms, sliced*

4 *carrots, thinly sliced diagonally*

1 *small tender celery stalk, thinly sliced diagonally*

½ *small red cabbage, diced*

2 *scallions, greens included, sliced*

4 *T natural soy sauce*

1. Heat the oil in a large skillet. Add the onion, reduce heat, cover, and cook slowly until tender, about 15 minutes. Do not allow the onion to darken.

2. Add all the other vegetables and cook, covered, for 5 minutes. Add the soy sauce and cook until the vegetables are just tender. Serve over brown rice or couscous, with whole wheat noodles, or over mashed potatoes.

CARROTS WITH ONION AND PARSLEY

Serves six

8 *medium carrots, peeled*

1 *tsp. cold-pressed olive oil*

½ *onion, quartered and sliced*

1 *clove garlic*

5 *parsley sprigs*

salt to taste

1. Cut the carrots into 2-inch pieces. Cut lengthwise to make sticks about ¼ inch thick. Steam for several minutes until the carrots are barely tender.

2. Heat the oil in a skillet. Cook the onion slowly until it is translucent. Don't let it brown.

3. Chop the garlic and parsley together. Add to the onions and cook for 1 minute more. Add the steamed carrots and salt and cook, covered, for 5 minutes.

13

SWEETS AND
OTHER TREATS

BANANA-STRAWBERRY
TOFU PUDDING

Serves six to eight

In Los Angeles there is a remarkable small chain of natural food markets known as Mrs. Gooch's. This recipe comes from their deli section where fresh, natural take-home is prepared daily.

2 16-oz. packages firm
  Chinese tofu, drained

1 C honey or unsweetened
  fruit juice concentrate

¼ C fresh lemon juice

1½ T finely grated lemon
  peel

1½ T natural vanilla

⅔ C grated fresh coconut

4 bananas, ripe but not
  brown, sliced

1 pint strawberries, ends
  removed, sliced

1 kiwi fruit, peeled and
  sliced for garnish

1. Combine the tofu, honey, lemon juice, lemon peel, and vanilla in a blender or food processor and blend until creamy and smooth. Add the coconut and blend for 1 minute more.

2. In a clear soufflé dish, layer the tofu mixture, bananas, and strawberries, reserving several strawberry slices for garnish. Top with the tofu mixture. Garnish with kiwi and strawberry slices. Chill 1½ to 2 hours.

AMARETTO MOUSSE

Serves eight

This dessert is so light and fluffy that it's hard to believe it contains no egg whites or whipped cream.

4 C mild soy milk or almond milk

⅓ C natural maple syrup

¼ tsp. salt

5 T arrowroot powder or kuzu

1 tsp. natural vanilla

2 T Pero or other powdered natural coffee substitute

1 T oil

2 T amaretto or kahlua

1. Place all the ingredients except the amaretto in a blender and blend at high speed for 3 minutes or until the mixture becomes very frothy.

2. Immediately place the mixture in a saucepan and bring to a boil over medium heat. Mix constantly with wire whisk or eggbeater, occasionally stirring with a spoon to prevent scorching.

3. Reduce heat and cook for 2 minutes more, stirring continuously. When the mousse has thickened, remove from heat and stir in the amaretto.

4. Chill, uncovered, in refrigerator for 2 hours.

NOTE. To make mousse pie, pour the mousse into a baked graham cracker crust and chill.

CHESTNUT CREME PUDDING

Serves six

Creme de marron, or chestnut creme, is a tradition in France as a holiday dessert. This recipe is a variation of that dish.

1 *lb. raw white sweet potato*

1½ *lb. raw chestnuts*

2 *T maple syrup*

1 *tsp. vanilla*

3 *T raw almond butter* or *raw tahini*

½ *C soy milk*

6 *pecan halves*

1. Steam the sweet potatoes whole and unpeeled, until tender. Let them cool until they can be handled. Remove the peels and cut into chunks.

2. While the sweet potatoes are cooking, remove the leathery chestnut shells with a sharp knife (there is a fuzzy skin directly on the meat of the chestnut that will be removed later). In a large water-filled saucepan, boil the shelled chestnuts for about 10 minutes or until they are tender and sweet. The best way to tell if they are done is to break off a small piece, peel it, and taste it. Pour out cooking water and cover chestnuts with cold water until they are cool enough to handle. A few ice cubes in the water speeds up the process. Remove the skins.

3. Place all the ingredients, except the soy milk and pecan halves, in a food processor and blend at medium speed. The mixture will be thick. Add the soy milk a little at a time until the texture is creamy. Don't add too much, even if you have some left over, or the chestnut creme will be too thin. Add more soy milk if necessary. Pour into individual dessert dishes, place a pecan on each, and chill at least 2 hours before serving.

ALMOND-ORANGE PUDDING

Serves six

1 *C blanched (shelled and skinless) almonds*

4 *C water*

⅛ *tsp. salt*

⅔ *C dry cream of wheat*

3 *T honey*

1 *T grated fresh orange rind (from ½ orange)*

1½ *T fresh orange juice*

1 *tsp. vanilla*

1 *T raw tahini, or Almond Butter (page 90), or Cashew Butter (page 89)*

6 *almonds*

6 *orange slices (from ½ orange)*

1. Mix the almonds and water in a blender or food processor at high speed until smooth, approximately 5 minutes.

2. Bring the almond mixture and salt to a boil in a saucepan. While stirring, add the cream of wheat, honey, and orange rind. Bring to a boil, reduce heat, and simmer, covered, for 15 minutes, stirring occasionally.

3. Remove from heat. Mix the fresh orange juice, vanilla, and tahini. After the cream of wheat has cooled for 2 minutes, stir in the orange juice mixture.

4. Pour into individual custard dishes and refrigerate, uncovered, for 2 hours.

5. Just before serving, turn out into individual dessert dishes and garnish each with an almond on the top and an orange slice on the side.

CASHEW PUDDING

Serves six

1 C raw cashews

3½ C water

4 T arrowroot or *kuzu*

½ C maple syrup

1 T malt syrup

¼ tsp. salt

1½ tsp. natural vanilla
flavoring

dash natural butterscotch
flavoring (optional)

1. Place the cashews and water in a blender and blend at high speed for 5 minutes. Strain the liquid through a very fine sieve or double thickness of damp cheesecloth and discard the pulp. Blend again.

2. Mix the arrowroot with 4 tablespoons of cashew liquid until creamy. Place all the ingredients in a blender at high speed until frothy, about 3 minutes.

3. Bring all the ingredients to a boil in a medium saucepan, stirring constantly. Cook for 2 minutes longer. Chill and serve with Vanilla Refrigerator Cookies (page 238).

VARIATION. For an Almond Pudding, use 1 cup of Almonds instead of the cashews.

MACADEMIA NUT–MAPLE COOKIES

Makes 25 to 30 cookies

¼ C cold-pressed vegetable oil

½ C natural maple syrup

1½ tsp. natural vanilla flavor

2 C whole wheat pastry flour

1½ tsp. baking powder

dash of salt

½ C chopped macademia nuts or pecans

1. In a bowl, combine the oil, maple syrup, and vanilla and whisk until creamy.

2. Mix the flour, baking powder, and salt and sift into the maple syrup mixture. Mix well with a wooden spoon until smooth. Add the chopped nuts and mix well.

3. Preheat the oven to 350°F. Drop teaspoon-size portions onto an oiled baking sheet, keeping the cookies about 1½ inches apart. Bake for 12 minutes.

RASPBERRY SCOTTISH SHORTBREAD

Makes 16 bars

⅔ C whole wheat pastry flour

½ tsp. salt

3 C raw quick-cooking oatmeal

⅔ C less 1 T cold-pressed vegetable oil

½ C less 1 T natural maple syrup

2 tsp. vanilla

½ C fruit-only raspberry jam

1. Sift the pastry flour and salt into the dry oatmeal.

2. Add the oil to the dry ingredients, and mix well.

3. Add the maple syrup and vanilla and mix thoroughly.

4. Preheat the oven to 350°F. Lightly oil a 9-by-9-inch baking pan. Cover the bottom of the pan with half of the batter, pressing firmly into place with fingers. Spread the jam evenly over the batter to cover. Cover with remaining batter. Press gently with your fingers to pack it in tightly and bake for 35 minutes. Cool 15 minutes and cut into bars.

GRANOLA BARS

Makes 12 bars

¼ C unsulfured raisins

1 T apple juice

1 C old-fashioned rolled oats

¼ C fresh wheat germ

¼ C roasted peanut pieces

¼ C shredded coconut

2 T cold-pressed vegetable oil

2 T malt syrup

1 T maple syrup or honey

3 T peanut butter

1. In a small skillet heat the raisins and apple juice. Bring to a boil, turn off the heat, cover, and let stand until raisins are plump.

2. Combine the oats, wheat germ, peanuts, and coconut. Add the raisins and mix well with your fingers to make sure that the fruit does not stick together.

3. Heat the oil, malt syrup, and maple syrup, stirring until it becomes liquid. Remove from heat and stir in the peanut butter.

4. Pour the syrup mixture over the dry ingredients and mix well with your hands.

5. Preheat the oven to 300°F. Pour the batter into a 9-by-13-inch loaf pan lined with lightly oiled aluminum foil or parchment. Press down firmly on batter with the bottom of a small glass. Bake for 20 minutes, cool for 10 minutes, and cut into bars.

Vanilla Refrigerator Cookies

Makes 30 cookies

1½ C pastry flour

1 tsp. baking powder

⅛ tsp. salt

¼ C honey or maple syrup

2 T malt syrup

¼ C cold-pressed corn oil

1 tsp. natural vanilla

1. Sift the flour, baking powder, and salt together.

2. Whisk together the honey, malt syrup, and corn oil until creamy. Add vanilla and whisk. Add the flour and stir well to mix.

3. Refrigerate the dough for 30 minutes. Cut the dough into two parts. Roll into ropes about 1 inch in diameter, roll in waxed paper, and refrigerate for 3 hours or overnight.

4. Preheat the oven to 350°F. Slice the chilled dough and arrange on a baking sheet about 1½ inches apart. Bake for about 10 minutes or until the cookies start to turn golden.

Pinwheel Cookies

Vanilla Refrigerator Cookie batter (steps 1 and 2; page 238)

2 T carob powder

1. When the batter is mixed, divide into two equal parts. Add the carob powder to one part and mix well. Refrigerate both parts for 30 minutes.

2. On a lightly flowered board, roll out each section of dough to form two rectangles about ¼ inch thick.

Place the carob dough on top of the light-colored dough and roll up tightly. Wrap in waxed paper and refrigerate for 3 hours or overnight.

3. Preheat oven to 350°F. Slice the chilled dough and arrange on a baking sheet about 2 inches apart. Bake for about 10 minutes or until the cookies start to turn golden.

DATE-PECAN COOKIES

Makes 24 cookies

1 C whole wheat pastry flour

4 T date sugar (ground dried dates)

⅛ tsp. salt

½ tsp. baking powder

½ C coarsely chopped pecans

2 T cold-pressed vegetable oil

1 tsp. natural vanilla extract

4 T natural maple syrup

3 T mild soy milk

1. Combine the flour, date sugar, salt, baking powder, and pecans and whisk together to fluff the flour and mix the ingredients. Combine the oil, vanilla, maple syrup, and soy milk and whisk until creamy.

2. Pour the liquid ingredients into the center of the flour and stir with a wooden spoon until mixed.

3. Preheat the oven to 350°F. Moisten your hands slightly and form balls about 1 inch in diameter. Place 1 inch apart on a lightly oiled baking sheet and bake for 10 minutes.

SHORTCAKE

Serves six to eight

1½ C whole wheat pastry flour

2 T soy flour

2 T arrowroot powder

3 tsp. baking powder

¼ tsp. salt

⅓ C natural maple syrup

2 T cold-pressed vegetable oil

⅓ C soy milk

2 T Almond Butter (page 90) or Cashew Butter (page 89)

2 T fresh lemon juice

1 T grated coconut

1. Sift together the pastry flour, soy flour, arrowroot powder, baking powder, and salt.

2. In a mixing bowl whisk together the maple syrup and oil until creamy. Add the soy milk, Almond Butter, lemon juice, and grated coconut and whisk or beat with an eggbeater until frothy. Slowly stir in the flour.

3. Preheat the oven to 375°F. Pour batter into a lightly oiled, floured cake pan and bake for 30 minutes. Cool for 10 minutes and turn out onto a platter to finish cooling. Use for strawberry shortcake, serve dry with coffee or tea, or ice with Flamingo Frosting (page 259) or Coconut-Mocha Cream Frosting (page 260).

STRAWBERRY SHORTCAKE

Serves six

2 pints ripe strawberries

1 Shortcake (page 240)

½ C raw honey

1. Wash the strawberries and gently rub away seeds. Set aside one whole strawberry. Remove green tops of the rest and slice lengthwise.

Cover with honey and mix gently. Refrigerate for 1 hour.

2. Gently brush any crumbs off the top of the shortcake and cover with the strawberries. Garnish with the whole strawberry.

BASIC DESSERT CAKE

Makes 1 9-inch cake. Double this amount for a two-layer cake.

1½ C whole wheat pastry
   flour

2½ tsp. baking powder

¼ tsp. salt

6 T date sugar (dried,
   ground dates)

1½ C soy milk

1 T cold-pressed vegetable
   oil

¼ tsp. cream of tartar

2 tsp. vanilla

1. Sift together the flour, baking powder, and salt. Grind the date sugar into a finer powder in a mortar and pestle and stir into the flour.

2. In a mixing bowl, combine the soy milk, oil, cream of tartar, and vanilla and beat with an eggbeater for several minutes, until the mixture becomes thick and foamy.

Gently stir this mixture into the flour.

3. Preheat the oven to 350°F. Pour the batter into an oiled and floured 9-inch cake pan. Bake for 25 minutes or until a clean probe inserted into the center comes out clean. Frost with Flamingo Frosting (page 259) or Coconut-Mocha Cream Frosting (page 260).

APPLE LAYER CAKE

Serves eight

CAKE

1½ C whole wheat pastry
　flour

2½ tsp. baking powder

¼ tsp. salt

6 T date sugar (ground
　dried dates)

1½ C mild soy milk

1 T cold-pressed vegetable
　oil

¼ tsp. cream of tartar

2 tsp. natural vanilla

1 apple, peeled, cored, and
　grated

APPLE TOPPING

2 apples, peeled, cored, and
　finely chopped

½ C apple juice

2 T date sugar (ground
　dried dates)

¼ tsp. cinnamon

¼ tsp. cloves

1 T whole wheat pastry
　flour

RAISIN FILLING

1 C raisins

¾ C apple juice

1 T date sugar

grated rind of ½ lemon

1 T whole wheat pastry
　flour

½ C finely chopped walnuts

1. Preheat the oven to 350°F. To make the cake, mix 1½ cups of flour, the baking powder, salt, and 6 tablespoons of date sugar and whisk to aerate. Combine the soy milk, oil, cream of tartar, and vanilla in a separate bowl and beat for about 5 minutes or until the liquid becomes frothy and approximately doubles in volume. Gradually add the flour mixture to the whipped soy milk, stirring gently with a wooden spoon until the flour is completely combined. Gently stir in the grated apple. Pour the batter into an oiled and floured 9-inch cake pan and bake for 25 minutes or until a probe inserted into the center comes out clean. Cool the cake before removing it from the pan.

2. For the topping, in a saucepan combine the chopped apples, ½ cup of apple juice, 2 tablespoons of date sugar, cinnamon, and cloves. Boil, reduce heat, and cook until the apples are tender. Sprinkle in 1 tablespoon of flour, stirring briskly, and

cook for 1 minute more until the sauce has thickened.

3. For the filling, in a saucepan combine the raisins, ¾ cup of apple juice, 1 tablespoon of date sugar, and lemon rind. Boil, reduce heat, and cook until the raisins are plump. Sprinkle in 1 tablespoon of flour, stirring briskly, and cook for 1 minute more. Stir in the walnuts.

4. With a sharp, moistened bread knife, using a light sawing motion, cut the cake into 2 9-inch round layers. Retain 2 tablespoons of the raisin filling and spread the rest evenly on the first cake layer. Cover with the other layer. Spread the apple topping over the second layer and place the extra raisin filling in the center to garnish. Chill.

ITALIAN CHEESECAKE

Serves six to eight

20 *oz. firm Japanese tofu*

1 *lb. Chinese tofu*

Grated rind of one lemon

½ *C malt syrup*

1½ *tsp. fresh lemon juice*

2 *T cold-pressed vegetable oil*

2½ *tsp. natural vanilla extract*

dash of salt

3 *T pine nuts*

2 *slices unsulfured dried pineapple, chopped*

1 *unbaked Graham Cracker Crust (page 258)*

1. Preheat the oven to 350°F.

2. Combine all the ingredients except the pine nuts, dried pineapple, and crust in a food processor or blender and beat for 2 minutes or until smooth.

3. Stir in the pine nuts and pineapple.

4. Pour the mixture into the graham cracker crust and bake for 45 minutes or until a knife inserted into the center comes out clean.

APPLE PIE

1 9-inch covered pie

The most important thing in apple pie is the apples. Your pie will be only as delicious as your apples, so pick the tastiest ones.

5 apples, peeled and thinly sliced

1 T arrowroot powder

½ C date sugar (ground dried dates)

¼ tsp. cinnamon

dash salt

Whole Wheat Pie Crust, Double (page 258)

½ tsp. vegetable oil

1 tsp. honey dissolved in ½ tsp. water

1. Combine the apples, arrowroot, date sugar, cinnamon, and salt in a bowl and toss until the apple pieces are completely coated.

2. Follow steps 1 through 3 for Whole Wheat Pie Crust, Double. Brush the inside of the crust lightly with oil to prevent it from becoming soggy.

3. Turn the apples out into crust and shake gently back and forth to settle the apples.

4. Preheat the oven to 450°F. Roll out and place the upper crust according to the instructions. Crimp edges to seal, making a lip all around. Prick the top of the crust several times to allow the steam to escape.

5. Bake for 10 minutes. Reduce the heat to 350°F and bake for 40 minutes more or until the crust starts to brown.

6. Remove from the oven and brush the top with dissolved honey glaze.

BANANA CREAM PIE

CRUST

1¼ C graham cracker
crumbs

2 T cold-pressed vegetable
oil

1 T water

FILLING

3 T arrowroot powder

1½ C mild soy milk

1½ T honey or natural
maple syrup

4 T shredded coconut
(optional)

2 tsp. natural vanilla
flavoring

3 ripe bananas (not dark)

juice of ½ lemon

1. Preheat the oven to 350°F. Mix well all of the crust ingredients. Press firmly into a 9-inch pie pan. Crumbs should cover the bottom and sides but not the rim. Bake for 5 minutes.

2. To make the filling, combine all of the filling ingredients, except the bananas and lemon juice, in a blender and blend into a cream for 3 minutes. Transfer the ingredients to a saucepan. Bring to a boil, whisking constantly, lower the heat, and cook for 3 minutes, continuing to whisk. Cool for 15 minutes.

3. While the cream is cooling, slice two bananas and arrange them evenly over the bottom of the crust. Cover the bananas with the cooled cream.

4. Slice the remaining banana. Sprinkle with lemon juice and toss until the slices are coated to prevent darkening. Arrange the slices attractively on top of the cream. Cover and refrigerate for 2 hours before serving.

JAM TARTS

Makes 25 to 30 tarts

DOUGH

2½ C whole wheat pastry
    flour

¼ tsp. salt

4 T date sugar, (ground
    dried dates)

6 T cold-pressed vegetable
    oil

½ C ice water

⅓ C all-fruit natural jam

1. To make the dough, sift the flour and salt together into a mixing bowl. Add the date sugar and use a whisk to mix. Slowly mix in the oil and blend with a pastry cutter or forks. Sprinkle the ice water on the flour, a tablespoon at a time, and quickly mix in with forks.

2. Cut the dough into three equal parts. Place the dough between two sheets of waxed paper and roll into a rectangle about ⅛ inch thick. Cut into squares, 2 by 2 inches. Place about ½ teaspoon of filling in a diagonal line in the center of each square. Close the tart by folding over the two opposite unfilled corners. Have them meet in the center of the tart. Pinch them closed. Tarts will resemble little kites with jam showing at two ends.

3. Bake at 350°F for 20 minutes.

PRUNE TARTS

Makes 25 to 30 tarts

PRUNE FILLING
12 *sulfured pitted prunes*
1 *T fresh lemon juice*

water

Jam Tart dough (page 246)

1. Combine the prunes and lemon juice in a small saucepan with just enough water to cover. Bring to a boil, cover, and let stand for 1 hour or until prunes are plump and soft.

2. Press the softened prunes through a sieve, or mash in a food mill or ricer, adding soaking juice as you go.

3. Prepare the tart dough and fill with prune filling. Bake as directed.

PECAN TARTS

PECAN FILLING
¼ *C finely chopped pecans*
1 *T malt syrup*

dash of salt
¼ *tsp. vanilla*

Jam Tart dough (page 246)

1. Combine all of the ingredients for the pecan filling.

2. Prepare the tart dough and fill with the pecan filling. Bake as directed.

PEAR COBBLER

Serves six

6 *medium-size ripe pears*

2 *T arrowroot or kuzu*

1 *C apple juice*

2 *T apple juice concentrate or 1½ T honey*

dash of salt

½ *C crumbled walnuts*

2 *T cold-pressed vegetable oil*

¼ *C malt syrup*

¾ *C raw quick-cooking oatmeal*

⅓ *C whole wheat pastry flour*

1. Wash pears, cut them in half, remove the cores, and slice.

2. In a small saucepan combine the arrowroot with 3 tablespoons of apple juice and mix until smooth. Add the remaining apple juice, apple juice concentrate, and salt. Heat, stirring constantly, until the mixture becomes translucent and thickened, about 5 minutes.

3. In a large bowl combine the pear slices, walnuts, and arrowroot mixture and turn it out into a baking dish or casserole.

4. Preheat the oven to 350°F. Place the oil and malt syrup into the same small saucepan and heat until mixture is a thin liquid. Whisk to blend. Add the oatmeal and flour and stir until they are completely mixed with the syrup. Crumble the oatmeal mixture evenly on top of the pears. Cover with foil and bake for 25 minutes. Uncover and bake for 10 minutes more.

Fresh Berry Mold

Serves four (2 cups)

1 C filtered apple juice

1 T plus 1 tsp. agar flakes

1 tsp. to 1 T raw honey
(depending on how
sweet the strawberries
are)

1 pint (or a little more) ripe
strawberries

mint sprig

1. Pour the apple juice into a small saucepan. Sprinkle the agar flakes on top. Bring the apple juice to a boil and cook for 5 minutes, stirring once to incorporate the agar. Remove from the heat and stir in the honey. Let the mixture cool for 5 minutes.

2. While the apple juice and agar are cooking, wash the strawberries, rubbing gently with your thumb to dislodge as many seeds as possible.

Take five medium strawberries, slice them, and put them aside. Put the rest in a blender and purée until creamy, about 1 minute. Stir the blended strawberries into the apple juice mixture and stir in the sliced strawberries.

3. Pour into a mold or bowl and chill for 1 hour. Unmold onto a chilled plate and garnish with a mint sprig. If you like, serve with our Mock Whipped Cream (page 262).

DESSERT CREPES

Makes 10 crepes

Crepes are probably the best known of the elegant, traditional French desserts. Like so many French dishes, crepes usually use lots of eggs and butter. We have created tender, delicious crepes that use neither. Even though we usually recommend cooking on stainless steel or enamel, we make an exception in this case. In order to avoid the large amount of butter necessary to cook a thin crepe, we suggest a 7-inch nonstick coated skillet for the job, or a 7-inch stainless steel or enamel skillet coated with a very thin film of soy lecithin. We think it's a reasonable trade-off.

1 *T honey* or *maple syrup*
1¼ *C mild soy milk*
2 *tsp. oil*

¾ *C whole wheat pastry*
    flour
¼ *tsp. salt*

1. Put the honey in the soy milk and let stand about 10 minutes, stirring often to dissolve. Add the oil and whisk just enough to blend. In a separate bowl, sift together the flour and salt. Pour the soy milk mixture into the flour and stir just enough to mix. If there are any flour lumps in the batter, mix with a hand eggbeater for no more than 30 seconds. The batter will be smooth and quite thin.

2. Heat a 7-inch nonstick coated skillet so that a drop of water evaporates. Pour 2 to 3 tablespoons of the batter into the center of the pan. Very quickly tip the pan in a circular motion so that the batter spreads and completely coats the bottom of the pan. Cook until the bottom of the crepe starts to brown, 1 to 2 minutes. You can check it by lifting the edge of the crepe and looking underneath. Loosen the crepe all around with a broad spatula, then move the spatula gently under the crepe and flip it over. Cook the second side until it just starts to brown, about 2 minutes more. Serve immediately or cook up to 1 hour in advance and stack on a plate, cover, and keep warm. Crepe making takes a little getting used to, so try making the first batch for yourself!

ORANGE-BRANDY CREPES

1 *batch of Dessert Crepes (page 250)*

⅓ *C natural orange marmalade*

5 *orange slices*

SAUCE

3 *T honey*

2 *T brandy*

2 *T fresh-squeezed orange juice*

Spread each crepe generously with marmalade and roll it up. Place two on a dessert plate. To make the sauce, mix the honey, brandy, and orange juice. Heat just enough to dissolve the honey. Do not boil. Sprinkle 2 teaspoons of warm sauce over each crepe and garnish with orange slices.

CRANBERRY-APPLE COMPOTE

Serves six

Don't be fooled by the simplicity of this dish. It's a special treat all by itself for dessert, spooned over shortcake, in a nut butter sandwich, or as an after-school snack.

6 *sweet apples*

1 *package* (10 oz.) *raw cranberries*

1 *C apple juice concentrate*

1 *C natural apple juice*

1. Peel, core, and dice the apples.

2. In a saucepan combine the prepared apples, cranberries, apple juice concentrate, and apple juice. Cook over medium heat for 7 minutes. Mash with a hand masher.

PINK APPLESAUCE

Makes 3 cups

6 *red apples*   ¾ *C natural apple juice*

1. Peel four of the apples, but core and dice all of them. The red peel of the two unpeeled apples gives the sauce its pink color.

2. Combine the apples and juice in a saucepan. Cook for 7 minutes, then cool for 15 minutes and purée in a blender or food processor.

FROZEN POPS

Although you can make frozen pops in your ice trays by using plastic spoon handles as the sticks, we have found that the plastic molds made for this purpose that are sold in supermarkets are the best. Each stick has a built-in tray for catching melting juice.

Pour fresh, unsweetened juice into the molds, insert the sticks, and freeze for at least 4 hours. Allow warm water to run over the outside of the mold for a few seconds to loosen the pop.

VARIATIONS. Add a ripe banana or peach to the juice and blend until smooth in a blender and freeze as above.

Purée ripe fruit (peaches, apricots, berries, watermelon) in a blender until smooth and freeze as above.

STRAWBERRY DESSERT

Makes 1 pint

Besides being much lower in fat per serving than ice cream, this dessert has the advantage of not needing an ice cream maker. Your freezer will do the job just fine.

¾ pint of ripe strawberries

½ T to 1½ T honey (The amount of honey depends on the sweetness of the fruit and of the sweet tooth.)

½ C soy milk

1 tsp. cold-pressed vegetable oil

⅛ tsp. cream of tartar

1. Wash the strawberries and remove seeds by rubbing gently with fingers. Dry them off with a paper towel. Take two berries and slice them. Set aside. Cut up the rest of the berries and blend in a blender with the honey until they are creamy and a little frothy, about 2 minutes. Set aside.

2. Place the soy milk, oil, and cream of tartar in a bowl and whip with a hand mixer until the mixture forms mounds when brought up with a spoon or the beaters, about 10 minutes.

3. Continue to beat while slowly adding creamed strawberries. Beat for another 2 minutes.

4. With a spoon, stir in the sliced strawberries. Place in a covered container and freeze, stirring every half hour.

VARIATIONS. Try other fruit such as peaches, apricots, raspberries, boysenberries, blueberries, or papaya. Use about 1 cup of the coarsely cut fruit.

Refrigerate the dessert instead of freezing and use as a topping for fresh fruit, ambrosia salad, pancakes, or shortcake.

BANANA SPLIT

Serves two

This dessert is light and very pretty.

1 *large apple, peeled*

2 *T apple juice*

1 *large banana, peeled*

2 *T Nut Butter Sauce (page 260)*

2 *T chopped peanuts*

2 *fresh strawberries or raspberries*

1. Cut the apple in half and remove the core. In a saucepan, place the apple juice and then place the apples halves, flat side down. The saucepan should be just large enough to accommodate the apples and no larger. Cover and cook the apples at low-medium heat for 7 to 10 minutes or until they are tender. Do not allow the apples to overcook or they will collapse. Place each apple, flat side down, on a dessert dish and spoon on any juices that are left in the saucepan. Chill, covered, for 2 hours.

2. Cut the banana in half lengthwise and cut each piece in half through the middle. You will have four pieces of banana half as long and half as thick as the whole banana. Place two banana slices, side-by-side, flat side down, on each plate. With a spatula, lift each apple half and place it, flat side down, on top of the bananas. Spoon half of the butter sauce over each apple. Sprinkle the chopped peanuts over the sauce. Garnish with the strawberries or raspberries.

VARIATION. Substitute Tofu Fruit Sauce (page 261) for the Nut Butter Sauce and top with Mock Whipped Cream (page 262).

CAROB FUDGE

Makes 25 pieces

Dark, rich, creamy fudge. Who can resist?

½ C raw cashew pieces

½ C mild soy milk

½ C unsweetened carob chips

4 T malt syrup

1 tsp. cold-pressed vegetable oil

2 T grated coconut

⅛ tsp. salt

2 tsp. natural vanilla extract

2 T Almond Butter (page 90) or raw tahini

½ C chopped walnuts

1. Place the cashews and soy milk in a blender or food processor. Blend at high speed for 5 minutes. The mixture will be creamy.

2. Place the cashew cream, carob chips, malt syrup, oil, coconut, and salt in a saucepan. Bring the mixture to a boil, stirring. Cover and continue to boil over medium heat for 3 minutes. Remove cover and continue to boil, stirring occasionally, until temperature reaches 230°F on a candy thermometer, or until a small amount dropped into cold water forms a soft ball.

3. Remove from the heat. Let cool for about 15 minutes. Stir in the vanilla and Almond Butter and beat with a wooden spoon. Stir in the walnuts.

4. Pour out into a lightly oiled 9-by-9-inch baking pan and refrigerate, covered, for at least 2 hours.

MALT TAFFY

Makes about 20 candies

This candy is a must for Halloween and other holidays when a treat is called for. The treat starts when the kids get to help in the kitchen. Cashew Butter (page 89), peanut butter, or raw tahini can be used, but we prefer Almond Butter.

½ C malt syrup

4 T Almond Butter (page 90)

⅛ tsp. salt

1 tsp. natural vanilla extract

1. Measure the malt syrup in a lightly oiled measuring cup. Pour it into a small saucepan. Bring to a boil, and boil for 1 minute over medium heat, stirring constantly. Remove from heat and cool for 10 minutes.

2. Add the Almond Butter, salt, and vanilla extract and mix very well. The mixture will be very thick.

3. Turn out onto wax paper, and when it is cool enough to handle, knead and stretch it for 2 minutes (you won't have any trouble getting helpers for this part!).

4. Break off teaspoon-size chunks, and roll in 2-in-by-2-inch waxed paper squares, twisting paper closed at both ends.

GOVINDA'S HALVAH

Serves eight

This delicious confection, from Govinda's Natural Foods Restaurant in San Diego, California, is not a traditional halvah. It is easy to make and it does taste heavenly. We have substituted cold-pressed vegetable oil (not olive oil) in place of the fresh butter that Govinda's uses. It's a wonderful holiday treat. This dish is low in saturated fats and has no cholesterol, but it does contain a lot of unsaturated fat.

½ C cold-pressed vegetable oil

1 C farina (we prefer Arrowhead Mills Bear Mush)

¼ C broken walnut pieces

½ C plus 2 T water

½ C plus 1 T raw honey

1 tsp. natural flavoring (vanilla, maple, etc.)

½ C raw nuts (walnuts, pecans, or almonds)

1. Heat the oil in large frying pan or wok. Stir in the farina and cook over low heat for 25 minutes. Stir five or six times. Stir in the walnut pieces during the last 5 minutes.

2. In a saucepan boil the water. Remove water from heat, mix in the honey and natural flavoring, and stir into the farina. Cook over medium heat, stirring constantly, until the mixture thickens and balls up, about 5 minutes. Cool for 10 minutes.

3. While the farina is cooling, place the raw nuts in a blender or food processor and blend in bursts until nuts have the consistency of farina. When farina has cooled sufficiently for handling, knead in ground nuts. Form into a low cake and refrigerate for 12 hours. For a really festive look, press halvah into candy molds or form into balls using a large melon ball scoop and press a nut into the top. Chill.

Graham Cracker Crust

Makes 1 9-inch crust

1½ C graham cracker crumbs (Crumbs can be made by placing crackers between sheets of waxed paper and crushing with rolling pin or wine bottle.)

2 T whole wheat pastry flour

2 T oil

3 T water

Mix the ingredients well (try your fingers for this job) and press evenly onto bottom and side of pie pan but not onto rim. If the pie will be baked, fill the unbaked crust and follow directions for baking. If the pie will not be baked, bake the crust for 10 minutes at 350°F.

Whole Wheat Pie Crust, Double

Makes 1 covered 9-inch crust (cut recipe in half for a single pie crust)

It is important that all the ingredients and the bowl be very cold.

2¼ C whole wheat pastry flour

¼ tsp. salt

6 T cold-pressed vegetable oil

5 to 8 T ice water

1. Place all of the ingredients in the freezer for 1 hour before making the crust.

2. Sift together the flour and salt. Quickly cut in the oil using a fork or a pastry cutter. Flour should have the texture of cracked wheat. Quickly sprinkle on ice water, a tablespoon at a time, fluffing quickly with a fork each time. Add only enough water to allow the dough to hold together for rolling. Do not

overwork the dough or it will be tough.

3. Cut the dough into two parts, making one part a little larger than the other. Place the larger part between two sheets of waxed paper and roll into a circle about 1 inch larger than the pie pan, all around. Remove one sheet of waxed paper and invert the pie pan over the center of the dough. Place your hand under the dough and waxed paper and turn the pan right side up. Without removing the waxed paper, press the dough into place. Remove the paper.

4. Fill the pie.

5. Place the top crust between two sheets of waxed paper and roll out into a circle the same size as the pie pan. Remove one sheet of paper and place the dough, paper side up, on the pie. Remove the paper. Crimp the edges to seal. Make 4 holes with a sharp knife as vents. Bake as directed for the recipe you are using.

FLAMINGO FROSTING

Frosts 1 single-layer cake

5 T whole wheat pastry flour, passed through tea strainer to remove coarse bran

1 C natural apple-raspberry juice, or any natural, sweet red fruit juice

2 T cold-pressed vegetable oil

1½ tsp. natural vanilla

dash of salt

2 T raw honey

grated peel of ½ lemon

1. Combine the flour and juice in a small saucepan and bring to a boil, whisking constantly. If clumps appear, beat with an eggbeater until the mixture is smooth. Cook for 2 minutes or until the flour is thick. Cool for 15 minutes.

2. Combine the flour mixture and all the other ingredients in a blender and blend at medium speed until smooth. Cool for 30 minutes and whisk before frosting a cake or muffins. This frosting can also be used as a cake filling, and in place of syrup on pancakes.

Coconut-Mocha Cream Frosting

Frosts 1 single-layer cake

5 T whole wheat pastry
   flour
1 C soy milk
2 T cold-pressed vegetable
   oil
¼ tsp. salt

2 tsp. natural vanilla
3 T maple syrup
½ C macaroon coconut
1 tsp. carob powder
1 tsp. Pero or *other*
   powdered coffee
   substitute

1. Combine the flour and soy milk in a small saucepan and bring to a boil, whisking constantly. If lumps appear beat with an eggbeater until smooth. Cook for 2 minutes, stirring constantly, or until the flour is thickened. Cool for 15 minutes.

2. Place the flour mixture and all the other ingredients in a blender and blend at medium speed until very smooth. Cool for 30 minutes. Whisk well before using.

Nut Butter Sauce

Use this sauce as a topping over ice cream, puddings, and pancakes. Cashew butter (page 89) or raw tahini can be used, but we prefer Almond Butter.

½ C natural maple syrup
1 T Almond Butter (page
   90)

⅛ tsp. salt
½ tsp. natural vanilla
   extract

1. Boil the maple syrup, uncovered, in a small saucepan for 3 minutes. Transfer to a small mixing bowl and cool for 15 minutes. (Omit

this step for a more liquid sauce, which is better for pancakes, French toast, and waffles.)

2. Add all the other ingredients to the maple syrup and mix well with a wire whisk. Serve chilled as a dessert topping or unchilled as a pancake topping.

VARIATION. To make a Brandy Sauce, add 1 teaspoon brandy *or* dark rum.

TOFU FRUIT SAUCE

Makes 1 cup

This sauce complements breakfast crepes, cakes, and fresh fruit.

5 oz. Japanese-style tofu (soft)

½ C natural, fruit-only jam such as strawberry, cherry, apricot, peach, or berry

2 tsp. fresh lemon juice

pinch of salt

1 T honey

Place all the ingredients in a blender and blend until smooth. Refrigerate. Serve over blintzes, crepes, fruit salads, shortcake, and as a filling for layer cake.

MOCK WHIPPED CREAM

Makes about 1½ cups

Our pretend whipped cream whips up like the real thing, can be made a couple of hours in advance and refrigerated, and will crown your best desserts with richness and elegance. What it won't do is add gobs of fat to your diet, since it has only about one-third as much fat as the real thing.

½ C mild soy milk

½ tsp. agar flakes

1 T water

2 tsp. cold-pressed vegetable oil

⅛ tsp. cream of tartar

1 tsp. vanilla

1 tsp. to 1 T honey

1. Mix the soy milk, agar, and water in a small saucepan and bring to a boil. Simmer, covered, for 5 minutes until the agar has dissolved. Stir twice. Pour the soy milk mixture into a measuring cup and add just enough water to make ½ cup. Refrigerate for 45 minutes.

2. Combine the chilled soy milk mixture with the oil, cream of tartar, and vanilla and beat at high speed with an electric eggbeater. After about 3 minutes, slowly add the honey. Total whipping time is about 10 minutes. Cream will form into gentle peaks. Serve over fresh fruit or anywhere you would use real whipped cream.

NUT CREAM

Makes 1 cup

Try this topping over pancakes, shortbread, winter fruits, plain toast, or pumpkin pie.

½ C blanched almonds or cashews

½ C water

¼ tsp. salt

1 tsp. natural vanilla

1 T natural maple syrup or ¾ T honey

2 tsp. cold-pressed vegetable oil

1. Place the nuts and water in a blender and blend at high speed until they turn into a cream that is smooth, not gritty, about 10 minutes. Add all the other ingredients and blend for 30 seconds.

2. Refrigerate for 2 hours. Before serving, whip with an eggbeater for 1 minute. Nut cream will now have the consistency of a thick light sauce.

STRAWBERRY-ALMOND MILK SHAKE

Serves two

8 large ripe strawberries

1 ripe banana (not overripe)

2 C Raw Nut Milk (page 264)

2 strawberries for garnish

1. Wash 8 strawberries and gently rub away the seeds.

2. Place washed strawberries, banana, and Almond Milk in a blender and blend at medium speed until creamy. Chill and blend again for 1 minute just before serving. Put a cut in the 2 strawberries and straddle one on the edge of each glass.

RAW NUT MILK

Makes 1 quart

This delicious substitute for milk can be made from raw nuts such as blanched almonds, cashews, hazelnuts, or macadamias (very expensive). Because of its flavor, we find that almond milk is the most versatile. Use raw nut milk whenever milk is called for in a standard recipe.

1 C raw nuts (almonds should be blanched)

3½ C water

2 tsp. cold-pressed vegetable oil

1 T raw honey

dash of salt

Blend all of the ingredients in a blender at medium speed for 5 minutes. Strain through a very fine sieve or a double layer of damp cheesecloth and press all of the liquid out of the pulp. Reserve pulp for use in soups. Chill nut milk.

14

MEAT—WE CAN
LIVE WITHOUT IT!
HERE'S WHY

By Ariane

In the course of writing this book, Lindsay and I accumulated a lot of information on health and the environment. We had many discussions on whether or not to include it in this book. On the one hand, we felt it was important. On the other hand, we didn't want to foist it upon readers who were simply looking for a really great total vegetarian cookbook. This chapter is the solution. We have condensed the information and included it for those who are interested.

Educated, Medicated, Vaccinated, and Sick

In the United Nations 1987 Monitoring Report on population statistics, the table of life expectancies in developed nations ranks the United States in ninth place. On an average, Americans die younger than the Japanese, the Australians, the Greeks, and most of the Western Europeans.

Interestingly enough, we lead the world in medical technology and quality medical facilities; we are among the most educated, medicated, and vaccinated of peoples; our food is hermetically sealed in sanitized packages—never touched by human hands. Our meat has never seen a fly and we have no public drinking water that was first used to wash animals and laundry.

Why are our health statistics poor? The answer is simple: While the old infectious diseases such as polio, tuberculosis, and smallpox have been virtually eliminated in this country, as in the other developed nations, degenerative diseases, which account for six out of the top ten causes of death in the United States, have gone up by 40 percent to 200 percent since the turn of the century. The good news is that these degenerative diseases, i.e., coronary heart disease, cancer, stroke, diabetes, and liver disease, are closely related to diet and, therefore, we can do something to prevent them.

The chief offenders in the modern American diet aren't the food additives with names too complicated to pronounce, although undoubtedly they play their part. The offenders, salt, sugar, fat, and the lack of fiber are the major components of processed and prepackaged foods and foods of animal origin, such as meat, poultry, fish, milk products, and eggs. Ironically, these foods also form the mainstay of the modern American diet.

Interestingly enough, we Americans are getting wiser and have cut way down on our use of salt and refined sugar, yet we're eating them more than ever before in history. The reason is that these ingredients are added in huge quantities to processed foods to enhance their taste. The chances are good that if you are eating food that is processed or prepackaged, it contains excess salt and/or sugar.

A common misconception is that "natural" sweeteners such as honey, natural maple syrup, molasses, fruit juice concentrate, and malt syrup are harmless. In reality, these sweeteners are simple sugars (also called simple carbohydrates) just like white sugar; they react in the same way and should be used sparingly. We do prefer the "natural" sweeteners as they tend to be less processed than white or brown sugar and they contain trace amounts of vitamins and minerals that are completely missing from refined sugars.

Health problems caused by overconsumption of simple sugars include obesity, dental cavities, and a rise in blood pressure, cholesterol, and serum triglycerides. The latter three are important contributors to heart disease. Laboratory tests have also shown that eating large quantities of sugar reduces the body's ability to fight infection. And, although the reason is not fully understood, further studies link high sugar consumption to alcohol abuse.

Another problem with refined sugar consumption is that sugar molecules are extremely small and need no digesting. They are simply absorbed all at once into the blood, causing a sudden rise in blood sugar. Most of us experience this as a "sugar rush," possibly along with some anxiety. This is followed by a sugar let-down, and often depression. Parents might notice an increase in out-of-control behavior in their little ones about twenty minutes after the children eat sugar. Children, who are more sensitive and often consume more sugar than adults, can become hyperactive and then depressed and withdrawn. Pediatrician Lendon Smith, in his book *Improving Your Child's Behavior Chemistry*, suggests that in many instances removing sugar from a child's diet will cure hyperactivity and other behavior problems including bedwetting.

Carbohydrates, whether simple (like sugar and honey) or complex (like grains and legumes), provide fuel for the body. Everything you do takes energy provided by carbohydrates. Unlike simple carbohydrates, though, complex carbohydrates are much slower to break down, and enter the bloodstream in measured amounts over a period of hours. They provide constant, dependable energy with no let-down. No wonder marathon runners prefer spaghetti to a steak or a brownie before a race.

When Better Is Worse: *The Real Skinny on Fat*

The new buzz words in health today seem to be *fiber* and *fat*. Experts agree that Americans consume only about half as much dietary fiber as required and about 50 percent more fat than is healthy. One reason is that Americans prefer protein from animal sources, which contains no fiber at all, and, in most cases, is very high in fat, rather than protein from high-fiber plant sources such as grains and legumes. We are eating half as much plant protein as our grandparents did and laxative sales vouch for the results.

Of the grains that we do eat, most have had their valuable fiber (as well as the vitamin- and mineral-loaded germ) processed out. The most common grains in our diet are wheat and rice, which finally reach us in the form of refined white flour and its products and white rice, respectively. Almost all of the crackers, breads, cakes, pastas, and many breakfast cereals on the grocery shelves are white-flour products. You might have noticed that recent medical disclosures about the importance of dietary fiber have left breakfast cereal manufacturers scurrying to add the bran back into their products. Apparently the wisdom of simply using the whole grain in the first place still eludes them.

Fiber is essential because of the way in which the human intestines are made. The long length is perfect for extracting nutrients from a high-fiber vegetable mass. The fiber keeps the whole thing moving and also carries away the toxins and bloodstream wastes that have been dumped into the intestines.

On the other hand, when it comes to digesting meat, poultry, fish, dairy products, or processed foods, which contain little or no fiber, the long length is a drawback. Without the fiber to propel it forward, the mass becomes sluggish and can remain decaying in the intestines for days. Toxins are produced that are absorbed through the intestine wall into the bloodstream along with some of the waste headed for excretion. Too little dietary fiber has been linked to an assortment of intestinal diseases, including colon cancer.

It is almost impossible to discuss the decrease in dietary fiber without also discussing the increase in dietary fat. The two run hand-in-hand because, unless you're living on instant mashed potatoes and soft drinks, the decrease in one almost always leads to an increase in the other.

Ah yes, fat. Most of it is either saturated or loaded with cholesterol, and it is in almost every bite we take. The short-term consequence of this dietary indiscretion is often impaired digestion, and all the discomfort that goes along with it. In the long run, there is obesity and possibly cancer or diseases of the heart and arteries.

Fat seems to be everywhere in our diets, but the prime sources are processed and fast foods and animal products. Those tasty snacks, such as crackers and chips, can derive up to 80 percent of their calories from fat; whole milk and fast food hamburgers deliver 50 percent of their calories in the form of fat; and for many meats, cheeses, poultry, and some fish the percentage can be even higher.

America's favorite source of fat by far is beef. Since 1945, Americans have doubled their consumption of beef, and these days the cattle (just like a lot of us) are much fatter than they used to be. Gone are the days of lean, range-fed steers that got plenty of exercise roaming freely in pastures. Here are the days of feedlot cattle who barely move for the three months prior to slaughter, while they gorge on grains and soy to fatten them up for our tables and our arteries.

The object of all this fattening is for the meat to get the highest possible grading. Contrary to popular belief, the fatter the beef (or the distribution of marbling), the higher the grading, the greater the price. Hence "select" is moderately fatty and moderately priced; "choice" is very fatty and fairly expensive; "prime" is very, very fatty, very expensive, and deadly. In this case, it can be said that "better" is definitely worse.

The bright spot is that in the last couple of years Americans have responded to the message about dietary fat by cutting down somewhat on the amount of beef consumption. The beef industry has responded by making more "select" grade meat available, and in some areas has raised the price to make it comparable to "choice."

At this point you might wonder why you didn't collapse after eating your first greasy hamburger on a white bun with fries. The reason is that the damage done in this way is cumulative rather than instantaneous, with the effects becoming apparent only after years of abuse. Most degenerative diseases begin slowly and imperceptibly. Consider, for example, that according to some experts, 46 percent of all American men have the beginnings of coronary heart disease by the time they are twenty-four, but the symptoms generally do not appear until middle age. If you are an American man over the age of thirty-five, you have a 75 percent chance of severe artery blockage.

While we're on the subject of fat, did you know that some frozen diet entrées derive up to 54 percent of their calories from fat? (The amount of fat recommended by the Surgeon General is 30 percent and other experts recommend less than that.) The calories in these "diet" dishes are often kept under 300 simply by giving you less food. Calculating the percentage of fat in a food is simple. All you need to know is the total calories in the food and how many grams of fat are in it—standard information on packaged food. This information is also available in nutrition tables such as the *Nutrition Almanac*. Since 1 gram of fat equals 9 calories, multiply the grams of fat by 9 and that will tell you how many calories come from fat. Next divide the fat calories by the total calories and that will tell you what percentage of the food is fat.

Chemical Cuisine

The chemical evils lurking in meat and poultry for the most part fall into three main categories: antibiotics, steroids, and pesticides.

ANTIBIOTICS

Antibiotics are a booming business. Approximately thirty million pounds of nearly a hundred different kinds are produced each year in the United States. Only about 55 percent are consumed by people. The rest are routinely fed to cattle, milk cows, chickens, and hogs, even when not medically indicated, simply because antibiotics make them grow bigger at a faster rate and have fewer infections.

The first problem is that the meat and poultry industries are not alone in having benefited from the reckless use of antibiotics. Many dangerous bacteria also have done well. So well in fact, that due to the continuous antibiotic assault, many bacteria responsive to antibiotics have been killed off, leaving those which are immune to thrive and evolve into resistant strains. In 1982, a Harvard study indicated that cattle in at least twenty states were infected with these resistant bacteria. When the Netherlands banned tetracycline, a common antibiotic, from use in livestock feed, the incidence of tetracycline-resistant Salmonella bacteria dropped by almost 60 percent in two years.

The second problem is that these resistant bacteria, primarily resistant Salmonella, are present in much of the meat and poultry, and some of the eggs we eat. If these foods are eaten without being cooked properly, the Salmonella bacilli are unaffected by the cooking process and live to take up residence in our intestines. The friendly intestinal bacteria confine Salmonella and similar infections to the digestive tract so long as we don't take any antibiotics. When we do, these helpful bacteria, which are not resistant to antibiotics, are weakened or completely destroyed and cannot prevent the Salmonella bacillus from passing through the intestine wall and winding up in the bloodstream.

The results of Salmonella infection can be severe. Experts estimate that from 270,000 to as many as 4 million people each year suffer from Salmonella poisoning. Some of these people are paralyzed or otherwise permanently disabled due to this infection and some die. And there is no improvement in sight. It seems as though we are headed to a time when the only cure for a bacterial infection will be a bowl of mother's soup and a hearty constitution.

STEROIDS

The accepted practice concerning the use of steroids or growth hormones is pretty similar to that of antibiotics. Steroids, too, are routinely administered to cattle to increase their bulk and shorten their fattening time. Interestingly enough, because steroids can be extremely dangerous, they are available to the human population only by prescription, or through the underground network that illicitly supplies them to bodybuilders and athletes who are willing to chance the side effects in order to acquire greater muscular bulk.

Use of steroids in animals is quite another story. Regardless of the fact that the steroids will eventually end up inside the people who eat the meat, there is very little regulation or enforcement of their use for livestock and poultry.

Steroids have wreaked some of the greatest mischief in the vulnerable little bodies of children. The most prominent effect of small doses seems to be the acceleration of the onset of puberty. Several years ago, in Puerto Rico, there was an epidemic of premature puberty in young children, with onset as early as four years old, in some cases. The cause was later traced by some researchers to the steroids and hormones contained in the meat, poultry, and dairy products that the children consumed.

There are measures before Congress, right now, which call for a ban on the use of steroids in some meat animals and a limiting of the use of antibiotics. The meat and poultry lobbies are fighting hard, and in an attempt to avert this kind of legislation they have started voluntarily cutting back on the use of steroids and antibiotics, but use of both is still common.

PESTICIDES

Unlike steroids and antibiotics, which are given directly to livestock, pesticides reach the animals indirectly as toxic residues in their feed. Although there are conflicting opinions on the long-term effects of pesticides on humans, one thing is known for certain: Nearly all of the pesticides consumed by an animal in its lifetime accumulate in its fat tissue and build up over time in increasing concentrations.

A piece of beef can contain up to twenty times more toxic chemicals than an equal amount of some vegetables. And that's saying a lot, considering the ridiculously large amounts of pesticide residues in our fruits and vegetables. When grain-fed beef or poultry is eaten, all the accumulated toxins in the meat are eaten right along with it. After the meat is digested many of the toxins are absorbed into the blood, and then stored in our fat. And except in the case of lactating mothers, where some of the toxins are passed on to their babies in their milk, the toxins will remain in the body, possibly for a lifetime. Some of these chemicals, including DDT, heptachlor, and dioxin, are extremely toxic and have been linked to cancer, birth defects, and death.

A Bad Investment:
The Environment Pays the Price

The diseases of the human body caused by an animal-based diet are the primary concern for most people. But there is another concern that is just as pressing even though it is invisible to most of us. That is the damage to the environment caused by the growing of animals for food. That is not to say that the use of resources for the production of meat is any more ruthless with the ecology than is agriculture and industry in general. It is just that the percentage of these taxed and depleted resources used to raise meat is so great, and the resultant nutritional yield is so puny, that it is an extremely foolish if not a downright dangerous investment. To put things into perspective, it is valuable to take a look at just how much of our natural resources are consumed by livestock and how much nutrition they provide in return.

According to the U.S. Department of Agriculture, of all the water consumed for any purpose in the United States, 50 percent goes to feed livestock. Over one-third of all the raw materials consumed for any purpose, including industry, and half of all the agricultural yield used domestically, is consumed by livestock.

This, in itself, would not necessarily be bad if we got most of it back in the way of food. But, sadly, this is not the case. Beef gives back only 10 pounds of edible protein for every 100 pounds of protein consumed, and only 4 calories for every 100 calories consumed. The numbers are similar for other meats and poultry and slightly better for eggs and milk. Said another way, fourteen vegetarians can live on the resources needed to feed only one person who eats meat and animal products.

Back when cattle roamed the range and ate wild grasses, getting back even 10 pounds of protein or 4 calories was a good deal. The rain fell and made the grasses grow. Neither rain nor grasses had any material value to humans and they cost nothing. Cattle roamed freely in the verdant pastures, turning plants that were not edible by humans into usable protein. Animal waste was dispersed over a wide area and eventually returned to the land to make it more fertile. In this way, cattle were protein factories and the equation made sense.

It was only when meat growers started bringing cattle in from pasture for fattening that the equation turned bad. Cattle do not need high-quality protein such as grains and soy, and when such feed is given to them, the animals become waste factories. With the efficiency of a bureaucracy they turn 100 percent high-quality edible protein into 90 percent waste and 10 percent edible protein.

THE CYCLE OF RUINATION

The subject is touchy because it deals with a part of American life that we hold sacred: farming. Fifty years ago most Americans lived on farms and the farm was where home was. But times have changed and the farmer and his land have fallen on hard times. Overproduction and overuse of natural resources have spoiled both farm ecology and farm economy and has pitched the farmer into a cycle of ruination.

THE 2,500-GALLON STEAK

The question of the availability of water is about as old as life: After all, it comprises most of the body weight of living organisms. Civilizations flourished where water was readily obtainable. Wherever there was civilization there was agriculture. For most of human history, agriculture depended on the generosity of nature to provide the rains and the regular flooding of the rivers. Humans waited while the waters came and went. When nature was stingy, humans went hungry. But this has changed. Sometime during this century we became impatient with nature and started helping ourselves to earth's hidden underground water reserves, called aquifers, in order to irrigate crops on land that until then had not been farmable. We could do this because, for the first time in history, we had the capability to produce the energy and the pumps necessary to remove huge quantities of water from the ground.

Aquifer water is millions of years old. It accumulates in the porous underground rocks slowly and it moves just as slowly. Unlike rivers and lakes, which swell and recede according to the seasons, aquifers are replenished so little at a time that in dry areas they can almost be considered nonrenewable. And therein lies the problem.

Every day in the United States we extract billions of gallons of water more than is replenished by rains and runoff. At the present rate of extraction, the Ogallala aquifer, which is the largest in the Unites States and supports half of the cattle produced in this country, could run dry in thirty-five years. By then, out of necessity, land being farmed will have been reduced by as much as 40 percent. For now, however, the water level drops while feed crops drink their fill. By the time it sizzles in the skillet, a one-pound steak has consumed 2,500 gallons of water, an egg has cost 120 gallons of water, and except for pumping costs, all of it is very cheap to agricultural businesses.

LIVESTOCK POLLUTION:
BEYOND THE GREENHOUSE EFFECT

While doing research for this chapter I read an article about the greenhouse effect, the global warming caused by the accumulation of certain atmospheric gases. Bovine belching and flatulence (escaping intestinal gas in cattle), it seems, was being considered as a possible cause of this atmospheric phenomenon. To the sober individuals who study the atmosphere this report must have originally come as comic relief. However, new evidence shows methane, the major component of digestive gas in livestock, to be an important element in the greenhouse effect. There are about one-and-a-half billion head of cattle on earth and each one releases a daily volume of gas greater than its body. These cumulative millions of cubic feet of gas enter the atmosphere to contribute to global warming.

To those studying earthbound pollution the problem is even more basic. It has to do with the colossal amounts of manure produced annually. Global warming notwithstanding, manure is the most problematic pollutant directly attributable to livestock themselves. Millions and millions of tons of it are heaped in mountains around feedlots where cattle are held for months to fatten. It is one thing to degrade manure dispersed over large areas of grazing land, and quite another to dispose of the prodigious amounts produced by the penned-up animals.

Initially, the heaps of waste affect mainly the farmer, who is faced with the formidable task of disposing of it—that is, where to put it all and how to get it there. Eventually, however, as the waste is washed into the water supply by rain, it becomes the problem of all the water users downstream. High concentrations of nitrates and nitrites, both of which are toxic, are produced by the degrading manure. According to Frances Moore Lappe in her book *Diet for a Small Planet*, cattle produce more harmful organic waste than all the human population and industry in the United States put together. And, so far, they receive little or none of the bad press or clean-up cost.

While cattle are directly responsible for the manure they produce, they are indirectly but no less responsible for the greater problem of chemical pollution, by virtue of what they eat. The chemical pollutants enter the ecology in the cultivation of livestock feed. Farmers, following package directions, apply staggering amounts of chemical fertilizers to crops, especially corn, which is responsible for 43 percent of the fertilizer use in the United States.

According to the USDA, 15 percent to 54 percent of the nutrients added to soil are not used by the plants but rather remain in the earth, eventually seeping into the groundwater and polluting it with nitrates, chemicals implicated in cancer. Where wells provide a substantial portion of water suitable for drinking, the pollutants quickly show up in the lemonade, coffee, and baby formulas of a large portion of the population. In Iowa, at least 20 percent of all the wells exceed federal limits for nitrates. At times when the amount of nitrogen fertilizers added to corn crops is increased, nitrate levels in well water increase by a proportional amount. In some wells, the concentration is high enough to cause birth defects, even death, in infants.

The fertilizers that are not used by the plants eventually find their way into streams, rivers, bays, and even our groundwater. In surface waters they do what they were designed to do: make green things grow. In most cases, the green things are algae, which are neither useful nor wanted in these waterways. Algae grows out of control, choking off natural vegetation, which is home for a vast variety of aquatic life.

Chesapeake Bay suffers from such a condition. Algae, nourished by agricultural runoff, have destroyed and replaced the plants where the once-thriving population of striped bass spawned. The striped bass are gone now and with them the fishermen who made their living there.

Although fertilizers and manure are major water pollutants, they are by no means the only agricultural residues found in groundwater. At least seventeen different pesticides and herbicides have been found in drinking water in at least twenty-three states and most are there to stay for a very long time. Since groundwater often travels only about one foot per year, and since at present we have limited technology for cleaning it up, this water could remain contaminated for thousands of years even if no new pollutants were to be added.

TOPSOIL EROSION: A LOSS WE CAN ILL AFFORD

The damage to the land itself comes in the form of topsoil erosion, whereby previously fertile farmland is laid bare by wind and rain. According to the USDA, the greatest contributors to erosion are feed crops, with corn alone responsible for 25 percent. Like groundwater, topsoil accumulates over a very long time. It takes thousands of years to create enough topsoil to make an area fertile for crops, but it can be blown or washed away in just a few years. In some agricultural areas, as much as one-third of the topsoil has already disappeared. According to the Worldwatch Institute, every one-pound steak has cost the erosion of thirty-five pounds of topsoil.

In areas where the soil is too badly depleted to produce an abundant harvest, the distressed farmer perceives as his only alternative the addition of large amounts of chemical fertilizers in an attempt to wrench high yields out of the dying land. With each season the elements plunder a little more of the soil's riches until finally all the topsoil is gone and only blowing dust and deserted farmhouses remain.

And while farmers lament the loss of valuable topsoil, others lament its accumulation: in waterways where it chokes off rivers and streams and reduces the capacity of lakes and reservoirs.

There are exciting alternative agricultural methods that would both preserve the ecology and allow for the raising of meat animals. This would involve rotating damaging crops such as corn with beneficial forage crops such as alfalfa and clover, which could be used to feed livestock. In doing this, the number of cattle that could be supported would decrease and ultimately the cost per pound of meat would rise substantially. Although meat would no longer be cheap, the shelf price would then reflect the real cost of meat. Meat is cheap only when the real cost in terms of water depletion, pollution, and erosion have not been figured into the final cost. At that point, we would see what a kick in the pocketbook meat really is.

OVERGRAZING: WHOSE PASTURE IS THIS, ANYWAY?

In the first draft of this section I omitted the problem of overgrazing. The other three problems were so monumental and pressing that overgrazing seemed almost incidental.

But I was wrong because it is now evident that the problem of where cattle are grazing can put the world out of business as quickly as pollution, water depletion, and erosion. The booming beef industry in Latin America, fueled by our seemingly insatiable appetite for fast food hamburgers, is responsible, to a great extent, for the burning of rain forests in Central and South America. This burning not only pours out millions of tons of greenhouse gases (which are gradually warming our atmosphere and may warm it sufficiently to cause drought, famine, and coastal flooding) but seriously reduces the amount of living rain forests, which cleanse our air of greenhouse gases and give us oxygen to breathe.

As millions of acres of rain forests annually turn into millions of acres of pasture for the cattle of a few wealthy people, thousands of species of plants and animals hang on the edge of extinction, and thousands of families who made their homes in the forests find themselves homeless and unable to feed themselves. Stripped of their homes, their livelihood, and their dignity, they become a burden on their fellow human beings.

A Parting Word

Archeological evidence indicates that the human race evolved as vegetarians, not as carnivores. According to UCLA professor Jared Diamond, man the hunter is a romantic myth and "big-game hunting contributed little to our food intake until after we had evolved fully modern anatomy and behavior." Early man was lucky to bag a rat or a bird or to steal a haunch from another animal's kill. For the most part, these early ancestors lived on the wild tubers, nuts, seeds, berries, and fruits they gathered. Meat- and animal-derived foods as a staple in the human diet are a recent innovation and one that neither our bodies nor the earth are equipped to handle.

When Lindsay and I became vegetarians, we each did so for our own health and the health of our loved ones. Over the years, though, we came to see that a diet that is not in harmony with nature causes problems on all levels of life: disease, environmental degradation, and the unspeakable suffering of food animals. In contrast, a diet that is in harmony with nature brings benefits to all levels of life: vital good health and beauty; an environment that gives us riches in abundance, sustains itself, and will graciously deliver its bounty to our children and to all future generations; and a global society where all inhabitants, whether human or animal, are treated humanely. When we saw how well we could eat on a diet that was in harmony with nature, it was clear to us that our choice was no longer only one of the intellect but also one of the heart.

Recommended Reading

Bennet, W., and J. Gurino. "Do Diets Really Work." *Science* 82:42–50, 1982.

Boslough, J. "Rationing a River." *Science* 81:26–37, June 1981.

Brown, M. "Here's the Beef: Fast Foods are Hazardous to Your Health." *Science Digest*, 31–36, April, 1986.

Cain, Carol. "The Calcium Hoopla." *Vegetarian Times*, 46–49, May 1987.

Cohen, L. C. "Diet and Cancer." *Scientific American*, 42–48, Nov. 1987.

Davenport, Horace W. *A Digest of Digestion*. Yearbook Medical Publishers, 1975.

Diamond, Jared. "The Great Leap Forward." *Discover*, 50–60, May, 1989.

Dickerson, J. W., G. J. Davies, and M. Crowder, "Disease Patterns in Individuals with Different Eating Patterns." *Journal of the Royal Society of Health* 105:191–194, 1985.

Dixon, B. "Overdosing on Wonder Drugs." *Science* 86:40–43, May 1986.

Fruhling, L. "Please Don't Drink the Water." *Progressive* 50:31–33, Oct. 1986

Goldwater, Leonard J. "Mercury in the Environment." *Sci. Am.* May 1971.

Grady, Denise. "Can Heart Disease Be Reversed?" *Discover*, 54–68, March 1987.

Hallberg, George R. "Agricultural Chemicals in Groundwater." *American Journal of Alternative Agriculture* II:3–13, Winter 1987.

Hardinge, M. G., and Hulda Crooks. "Non-Flesh Dietaries." *Journal of the American Dietetic Association* 43:538–558, Dec. 1963.

Hardinge, M. G., and F. G. Stare. "Nutritional Studies of Vegetarians." *The Journal of Clinical Nutrition* 2:73–82, Mar.–Apr. 1954.

Hopson, Janet. "A Key to Health in Performance." *Science Digest* 65–67, Jan. 1984.

Jensen, O. M. "Cancer Risk Among Danish Male SDA and Other Temperance Society Members." *Journal of the National Cancer Institute* 6:1011–1014, 1983.

Karliner, J., D. Faber, and R. Rice. "Nicaragua, An Environmental Perspective." *Green Paper.* The Environmental Project on Central America, 1986.

Kirschmann, John D. *Nutrition Almanac.* McGraw-Hill Book Company, New York, 1983.

Lappe, F. M. *Diet for a Small Planet.* Ballantine Books, New York, 1982.

Liebman, B. "Calories Don't Count . . . Equally." *Nutrition Action Health Letter*, Center for Science in the Public Interest, vol. 16, 8–9, Jan./Feb. 1989.

Little, C. E. "The Great American Aquifer." *Wilderness* 51:43–47, 1987.

Moser, Penny Ward. "It Must Be Something You Ate." *Discover*, 94–100, Feb. 1987.

McDougall, John A. *The McDougall Plan.* New Publishers, Piscataway, N. J., 1983.

Neiman, David C. "Vegetarianism: Nutritional Adequacy and Relationships to Health and Fitness." Loma Linda University, Loma Linda, Cal., 1986.

Palmer, S., and K. Bakshi. "Diet, Nutrition and Cancer." *Journal of the National Cancer Institute* 70:1151–1170, 1983.

Papendeck, Robert I., Lloyd F. Elliott, and James F. Power. "Alternative Production Systems to Reduce Nitrites in Groundwater." *American Journal of Alternative Agriculture* II:19–24, Winter 1987.

Peskin, H. "Cropland Sources of Water Pollution." *Environment* 28:30–34, 1986.

Phillips, R. L. and D. A. Snowdon. "Association of Meat and Coffee Use with Cancers of the Large Bowel, Breast and Prostate Among SDA." *Cancer Research* 43:48–51, 1983.

Register, U. D. et al. "Influence of Nutrients on Intake of Alcohol." *Journal of the American Dietetic Association* 61:159–162, August 1972.

Robbins, John. *Diet for a New America.* Stillpoint Publishing, Walpole, N.H., 1987.

Rogers, Pete. "Water: Not As Cheap As You Think." *Technical Review* 89:30–43, 1986.

Rolland, R. M. et al. "Antibiotic-Resistant Bacteria in Wild Primates." *Applied and Environmental Microbiology* 49:791–794, 1985.

Sanchez, A. et al. "Role of Sugars in Human Neutrophilic Phagocytosis. *The Journal of Clinical Nutrition* 26:1180–1184, Nov. 1973.

Sanchez, Albert, J. A. Scharffenberg, and U. D. Register. "Nutritive Value of Selected Proteins and Protein Combinations." *The American Journal of Clinical Nutrition* 13:243–253, 1963.

Sanders, T. A. B. "Strict Vegetarianism." *Advances in Diet and Nutrition.* London: John Libby & Co. Ltd., 1985.

Sapolsky, Robert M. "Junk Food Monkeys." *Discover.* 48–51, Sept. 1989.

Shell, Ellen Ruppel. "Snake Oil: Don't Believe Everything You Hear About Dietary Fat." *Atlantic*, pp. 74–75, August 1987.

Simpson, H. C. R., and J. I. Mann. "The Dietary Management of Diabetes." *Advances in Nutritional Research* 7:39–69, 1985.

Small, Margaret. "The Cholesterol Connection." *Science Digest*, p. 18, Feb. 1986.

Smith, Lendon H. *Improving Your Child's Behavior Chemistry*. Simon and Schuster, New York, 1976.

Woodwell, George M. "Toxic Substances and Ecological Cycles." *Sci. Am.* March 1967.

Zaridge, David G. "Diet and Cancer." *World Review of Nutrition and Dietetics* 48:196–212, 1986.

Ziolkowski, Heidi. "Groundwater—Our Unseen Resource." *Calypso Log, The Cousteau Society* 14:14–16, Feb. 1988.

"Common Ground." National Audubon Society and TBS Productions, 1987.

"Ebbing of the Ogallala." *Time*, pp. 98–99, May 10, 1982.

"Grazing on Public Lands." *Wilderness* 49(2), p. 2, sum. 1986.

"Is Sunny-Side-Up a Salmonellosis Haven?" *Sci. News*, April 16, 1988.

"New Bones to Pick About Osteoporosis and Calcium Supplements." *Discover*, p. 8, Oct. 1986.

"Position Paper on a Vegetarian Approach to Eating." *Journal of the American Dietetic Association*, 77, July 1980.

Soil and Water Resources Conservation Act., Final Program Report and Environmental Impact Study, USDA, 1982.

"Steroids Stir Mental Backlash." *Science News*, April 30, 1988.

"What It Takes to Get a Steak." *Science News*, 133, 153, Mar. 5, 1988.

World Population Trends and Policies, 1987 Monitoring Report. Dept. of International Economic and Social Affairs Population Study 103, United Nations, New York, p. 135, 1988.

Index

A Note About the Authors

LINDSAY WAGNER first achieved widespread fame as television's "The Bionic Woman." Since that time she has worked virtually nonstop in a host of projects, including *The Taking of Flight 847: The Uli Derickson Story, Callie & Son, The Incredible Journey of Dr. Mag Laurel, Scruples, Passions*, and the Academy Award-winning film *The Paper Chase*.

As a private person, Lindsay Wagner has made a study of the healing arts since age twenty when she faced possible surgery for a stomach ulcer. A friend recommended a holistic doctor, whose therapy not only helped her cure the problem herself, but also enabled her to understand and treat the underlying cause of the illness. This dedication to the exploration of human potential, the foundation of which nutrition and health play important roles, is also demonstrated in her first book, *Lindsay Wagner's New Beauty: The Acupressure Facelift*, published by Prentice Hall Press in 1987.

ARIANE SPADE was born in Lyon, France. She attended the University of Southern California and the University of California at Los Angeles to study physics, writing, and art. Before taking up writing as a profession, she was a science and health teacher and worked as a designer and artist. In the last ten years, she has also focused much of her time working for environmental preservation, ending world hunger, and the human potential movement. She lives with her husband and daughter in Woodland Hills, California.